Baillière's
CLINICAL
PAEDIATRICS
INTERNATIONAL PRACTICE AND RESEARCH

Baillière's

CLINICAL

PAEDIATRICS

INTERNATIONAL PRACTICE AND RESEARCH

Volume 2/Number 3
August 1994

Epilepsy

E. M. ROSS MD, FRCP, MFPHM, DCH
R. C. WOODY MD, MPH
Guest Editors

Baillière Tindall
London Philadelphia Sydney Tokyo Toronto

This book is printed on acid-free paper.

Baillière Tindall	24–28 Oval Road,
W.B. Saunders	London NW1 7DX

The Curtis Center, Independence Square West,
Philadelphia, PA 19106–3399, USA

55 Horner Avenue
Toronto, Ontario M8Z 4X6, Canada

Harcourt Brace & Company
Australia
30–52 Smidmore Street, Marrickville, NSW 2204, Australia

Harcourt Brace & Company
Japan Inc,
Ichibancho Central Building, 22–1
Ichibancho, Chiyoda-ku, Tokyo 102, Japan

ISSN 0963–6714

ISBN 0–7020–1862–7 (single copy)

Baillière's Clinical Paediatrics is published four times each year by Baillière Tindall.
Prices for Volume 2 (1994) are:

TERRITORY	ANNUAL SUBSCRIPTION	SINGLE ISSUE
Europe including UK	£80.00 (Institutional) post free £70.00 (Individual) post free	£27.50 post free
All other countries	Consult your local Harcourt Brace & Company office for dollar price	

The editor of this publication is Catriona Byres, Baillière Tindall,
24–28 Oval Road, London NW1 7DX.

Typeset by Phoenix Photosetting, Chatham.
Printed and bound in Great Britain by the University Printing House, Cambridge.

Contributors to this issue

HASAN AZIZ MB, FRCPE, MRCP, FCPS, Professor, Department of Neurology, Jinnah Postgraduate Medical College, Karachi, Pakistan.

FRANK M. C. BESAG MB, PhD, FRCP, MRCPsych, DCH, Medical Director, St. Piers Lingfield, St. Piers Lane, Lingfield, Surrey RH7 6PW: Honorary Consultant, The Maudsley Hospital, Denmark Hill, London SE5 8AZ: Honorary Senior Lecturer, Institute of Psychiatry, DeCrespigny Park, London SE5 8AF, UK.

COLIN D. BINNIE MA, MD, BChir, Consultant Clinical Neurophysiologist, Maudsley Hospital, London SE5 8AZ, UK.

CAROL S. CAMFIELD MD, FRCP(C), Professor of Pediatrics, Dalhousie University Medical School, Division of Child Neurology, IWK Hospital for Children, PO Box 3070, Halifax, Nova Scotia, B3J 3G9 Canada.

PETER R. CAMFIELD MD, FRCP(C), Professor of Pediatrics, Dalhousie University Medical School, Division of Child Neurology, IWK Hospital for Children, PO Box 3070, Halifax, Nova Scotia, B3J 3G9 Canada.

SHIRLEY V. HODGSON DM, FRCP, BSc, DORCOG, DCH, Senior Lecturer in Clinical Genetics, Department of Medical and Molecular Genetics, UMDS Guy's Campus and Honorary Consultant in Clinical Genetics, St Mark's Hospital, London, UK.

EUAN M. ROSS MD, FRCP, MFPHM, DCH, Professor, Department of Community Paediatrics, King's College School of Medicine, South Western Hospital, London SW9 9NU, and Paediatrician to King's/Maudsley Centre for Epilepsy, London SE5 8AF, UK.

NIALL V. O'DONOHOE MA, MD, FRCP(I), DCH, 43 Orwell Park, Rathgar, Dublin 5; Professor of Paediatrics, Trinity College, Dublin (retired): Formerly, Consultant Paediatric Neurologist, National Children's Hospital, Dublin 2 and Our Lady's Hospital for Sick Children, Dublin 12, Ireland.

RUBY H. SCHWARTZ MBBS, MRCP(UK), DORCOG, Consultant Paediatrician and Honorary Senior Lecturer, Paddington Green Children's Unit, St. Mary's Hospital, London W2 1NY and Central Middlesex Hospital, London NW10 7NS, UK.

CHRISTOPHER M. VERITY MA, FRCP, Consultant Paediatric Neurologist, The Child Development Centre, Addenbrooke's Hospital, Cambridge CB2 2QQ: Associate Lecturer, Clinical School, University of Cambridge, UK.

ROBERT C. WOODY MD, MPH, Pediatric Neurologist, El Paso, TX 79902, USA.

Table of contents

Preface/E. M. ROSS & R. C. WOODY   ix

1   Current issues in children's epilepsy   451
    E. M. ROSS

2   Classification of epilepsies in infancy, childhood and adolescence   471
    N. V. O.DONOHOE

3   Principles of genetic counselling in the childhood epilepsies   485
    S. V. HODGSON & C. M. VERITY

4   Paediatric epilepsy in developing countries   507
    H. AZIZ & R. C. WOODY

5   Non-pharmacological approaches to children's epilepsy   529
    R. H. SCHWARTZ

6   Febrile seizures   547
    P. R. CAMFIELD & C. S. CAMFIELD

7   Epilepsy, education and the role of mental handicap   561
    F. M. C. BESAG

8   Neurophysiological investigations of epilepsy in children   585
    C. D. BINNIE

Index   605

PREVIOUS ISSUES

Vol. 1, No. 1 1993
Child Abuse
C. J. Hobbs & J. M. Wynne

Vol. 1, No. 2 1993
The New Genetics
I. D. Young

Vol. 1, No. 3 1993
Arthritis in Children and Adolescents
T. R. Southwood & P. N. Malleson

Vol. 1, No. 4 1993
Transplantation
M. Broyer

Vol. 2, No. 1 1994
Coma
J. A. Eyre

Vol. 2, No. 2 1994
Current Issues in the Adolescent Patient
R. S. Tonkin

FORTHCOMING ISSUE

Vol. 2, No. 4 1994
Paediatric Gastroenterology
B. S. Kirschner & J. A. Walker-Smith

Preface

This book is written for paediatricians who care for children with epilepsy, particularly those who despair in keeping up to date in a subject that affects them all yet figures relatively little in the major national and international conferences that they struggle to attend. Great changes in paediatric epilepsy are taking place to the potential benefit of the affected child, parents and extended family. New drugs are being launched and parents appear in clinics clutching newspaper cuttings about them; television shows the results of new advances in surgery and few are too shy to ask for a brain scan. This work is neither intended to be a stand alone complete textbook; both Aicardi's and O'Donohoe's new editions of their monographs perform that function admirably and a multi-author volume is unlikely to do it as well, nor is it a reference volume for the few epileptologists who tend to meet regularly but tend to keep their knowledge to themselves. We hope it will be regarded as the written equivalent of a symposium in which authors from both sides of the Atlantic have been given the space to discuss areas where they have made advances in the understanding of and practice of epilepsy in a way that will inform clinical practice. The first chapter is meant to be an exception and a starting point for those new to the world of paediatric epileptology; it started life ten years ago as lecture notes for London medical students; subsequently it has matured on a succession of computers becoming a handout for Professor Aziz's postgraduate course in Karachi before being expanded to its present format.

We are most grateful to all the contributors who produced their manuscripts at record speed with so little pain to the editors and to Margaret Macdonald and subsequently Catriona Byres and Karen Grace for their editorial skills that so quickly turned them into this book.

E. M. ROSS
R. C. WOODY

1

Current issues in children's epilepsy

EUAN M. ROSS

The 1990s see great changes in the world of children's epilepsy. The subject is the focus of much thought; old assumptions are being swept away as new means of investigating brain function and anatomy become available. Advances in the understanding of the physiological and molecular basis of the epilepsies are discussed in depth in *Epilepsy—Models, Mechanisms and Concepts* edited by Schwartzkroin (1993), in the five volumes that have so far been published in the series *Recent Advances in Epilepsy* edited by Pedley and Meldrum (further volumes are published every 2–3 years) and in the regular specialist journals *Epilepsia, Epilepsy Research* and *Seizure*.

This opening chapter gives an overview of some of the outstanding issues, controversies and areas where confusion reigns, and points the way to further reading within this volume and elsewhere. It has been impossible to condense all these issues into a few pages, and some repetition and overlap with other chapters is unavoidable.

CHALLENGES IN PAEDIATRIC EPILEPSY

After many years of little new in therapeutics, a dozen radically new anti-epilepsy drugs have either been marketed or are at the late premarketing stage. It is essential that they be fully evaluated, their mode of action, indications and side-effects known. Their price, at least initially, will be up to 20 times higher than that of existing drugs, reflecting their high development costs. Large-scale collaborative studies, similar to those used in evaluating the treatment of conditions such as leukaemia, are needed in order to learn about their indications and effectiveness.

The role of epilepsy surgery is becoming much better defined and new techniques are being developed (Engel, 1994). At the same time the social and educational needs of children are being voiced more loudly and it is becoming necessary for paediatricians to work ever more closely with educational and social services. As a result of all these pressures the speciality of 'paediatric epileptology' is emerging. There are far too many children with epilepsy to be managed solely by paediatric neurologists; the need is for new thought to cascade rapidly from the research centres into every day practice. Much of this new information about epilepsy in childhood tends to be closeted in specialist circulation journals and conferences attended by the few with a

Baillière's Clinical Paediatrics—
Vol. 2, No. 3, August 1994
ISBN 0–7020–1862–7

special interest in epilepsy. This book is intended to make some of this information more accessible to paediatricians.

Understanding of the aetiology and thus prevention of epilepsy in childhood remains at an elementary stage. Part of the problem stems from difficulties in obtaining a good epidemiological handle on the condition—whom it affects and the influence of possible premorbid circumstances. This lack of knowledge stems in part from a paucity of modern whole-community studies that incorporate appropriate control or reference cases. There is a need to resolve outstanding disagreements over definition and classification of epilepsy in childhood, and to use—and where necessary refine—the international classification. O'Donohoe takes up this theme in Chapter 2 and expands it in his textbook (O'Donohoe, 1994), these, carefully read, should help to reduce confusion and standardize practice.

CHILDREN WITH EPILEPSY HAVE MULTIPLE NEEDS

Many children with epilepsy have multiple medical problems of which the seizures are but one component; their doctors require a wide knowledge of children's medicine and therapy as well as neurological expertise and must be 'generalists' as well as having specialized knowledge. The management of epilepsy in childhood lies at the cross-roads between general practice, emergency medicine, community and hospital-based paediatrics. The occurrence of a first fit causes untold anxiety to parents and carers. Most children in developed countries having their first fit will be admitted to hospital. Many, perhaps 70% of parents, think their child is dying and may have a powerful yet unjustified preconceived vision of epilepsy as a permanent, disabling condition that may herald a blighted future. They need a great deal of repeated accurate counselling and may be helped by the books specially written for parents listed at the end of this chapter. In developing countries the problems of diagnosis are similar but the high cost of drugs relative to income, long distances, limited availability of expert help and investigation compound the problem (see Chapter 4 by Aziz and Woody). Few receive adequate treatment and these children suffer even more than in the West from discrimination.

Untested hypotheses abound in paediatric epilepsy. Facts based on sound epidemiological study and clinical audit are needed to determine which aspects of management are beneficial.

A BRIEF HISTORY

The word 'epilepsy' has been used in varying forms from early writings of the ancient Arabian physicians. Hippocrates (460–375 BC) wrote clear descriptions of convulsive disorders (Reynolds, 1988). The principles of management of epilepsy given by Galen, however, fossilized thought until the early 19th century when French physicians began to make clinical sense of the epilepsies, explaining why so much nomenclature is French in origin. This leadership continues to the present day, exemplified by Aicardi's textbook *Epilepsy in Children* (1993) and *Epileptic Syndromes in Infancy, Childhood and Adolescence* (1992) edited by Roger et al from Marseilles. Rational drug therapy began with the introduction of bromides in the late 19th century and barbiturates in the early 20th century. Brain surgery for epilepsy began at the end of the 19th century. The development of human neurophysiology applied to clinical epilepsy can be ascribed to Hans Berger who demonstrated the human encephalogram in Germany in the late 1920s. Tempkin (1971) wrote the standard history of epilepsy *The Falling Sickness*; librarians should be asked not to discard Lennox and Lennox's two-volume textbook *Epilepsy and Related Disorders* (1960) which summarizes clinical practice up to that time.

EPILEPSY OR 'THE EPILEPSIES'?

Epilepsy is not a single condition but refers to many aetiologically different disorders that result in a huge variety of seizure types which can be described in many different ways. This poses a dilemma which is well illustrated by infantile spasms (*inter alia*), which can be described in at least five distinct ways:

- Clinical manifestation: infantile spasms or salaam attacks.
- Eponym: West syndrome (West described his son's spasms in the *Lancet* in 1841).
- EEG description: hypsarrhythmia.
- Structural pathology: a number of discrete aetiological factors are known, including tuberose sclerosis, but many cases reveal no underlying cause.
- Response to therapy: some patients are very sensitive to steroids; others hardly respond to any medication.

The same problem of description and classification runs right through the whole canon of epilepsy. Some forms are as clear-cut an entity as the different types of congenital cardiac disorder; others can be very difficult to differentiate. Widely differing brain insults or abnormality can result in similar types of seizure. Some forms of epilepsy occur for no understandable reason such as in childhood absence epilepsy with a 3-Hz spike and wave (dart and dome) EEG; others have clear-cut pathology that is revealed on brain scanning or can be diagnosed from external clinical features as in tuberose sclerosis.

It is best to use the term 'the epilepsies' rather than 'epilepsy' when referring to the problem in general. Do not allude to 'epileptics' but use the more humane term, 'people/children with epilepsy'.

THE NEED FOR DEFINITION

It can be difficult to draw conclusions from research reports because different authors use different definitions of the word 'epilepsy', making it impossible to know whether comparable conditions are being described. In general, febrile convulsions are excluded from the definition. As an illustration, Ross et al (1980) used the following in their population studies: 'More than one episode of altered consciousness, sensation or movement, primarily cerebral in origin, unassociated with infection, metabolic state or fever.'

But when did the first seizure occur?

The definition given above is becoming contentious and forms the basis for lively discussion in academic circles; it is logical to regard epilepsy as beginning with the first fit, yet often it is impossible to know in retrospect when seizures started to occur (Hart et al, 1990; Berg and Shinner, 1991). Does epilepsy start when the first fit actually occurs or when the insult that led to the first seizure began? The same occurs in many conditions; for example, myocardial disease starts long before the 'coronary' patient presents with chest pain. First fits may not be witnessed or witnesses may be confused and give an unreliable history. In Chapter 7 Besag shows, using an EEG-based system that counts seizure events and by the scrutiny of videotape, that witnesses tend to undercount seizures. Nocturnal seizures may be completely missed.

Epilepsy and not-epilepsy; confusing presentations and misdiagnosis are common

Forty per cent of those reported to have epilepsy by at least one doctor to the UK National Child Developmental Study were regarded by the authors as not having a definite diagnosis of epilepsy (Ross et al, 1980); other studies came to the same conclusion. Misdiagnosis can lead to needless and potentially harmful medication and restrictions which may have a devastating effect on self-esteem and, ultimately, on career and marriage prospects, particularly in cultures where epilepsy is seen as a particularly stigmatizing condition.

On rare occasions children are admitted to hospital with a history of seizures, yet the clinical manifestations do not ring true and the EEG and other investigations may repeatedly be normal. What are these episodes?

An instructive anecdote

A boy aged 10 years was admitted to a children's hospital in 'status epilepticus' which responded to intravenous antiepilepsy drugs. He was on leave from a residential hospital school where he had been admitted at the age of 5 years following two generalized seizures at home. His mother developed schizophrenia; his father was a long-distance lorry driver and could not make arrangements for the child's care. For the next 2 years he had no seizures; the EEG was 'mildly abnormal'. He then started to have frequent generalized seizures. He had a florid fit in the course of a professorial ward round and a film was made for teaching purposes. A registrar gained the child's confidence and the truth came out. These were learnt episodes, copied from other children; a kindly foster family was found and the 'epilepsy' melted away.

Message: Some children have both true seizures and an ability to mimic them.

For discussion. Is it pejorative and 'victim blaming' to use the term pseudo-seizure?

The diagnosis of epilepsy must be reserved for those who actually have the condition. Those who have learnt phenomena need accurate diagnosis and psychiatric help (Betts, 1990; Metrick et al, 1991; Buchanan and Snars, 1993).

Munchausen syndrome by proxy

This occurs where a parent or carer fabricates seizure symptoms in a child who is then at risk of needless investigation and medication. The key is the lurid and usually 'not quite in the books' nature of the seizures which are never seen by an independent witness. This can be an extremely difficult problem to diagnose and manage. There may have been an earlier history of genuine seizures witnessed by independent observers; the EEG may show mild or inconsistent abnormalities yet no further seizures are witnessed by anyone apart from the carer, who may even resort to inducing altered consciousness in their child as an attention-seeking device (Meadow, 1991).

Genuine seizures, but not due to epilepsy

Breath-holding, faints, emotional outbursts, cardiac arrhythmia, syncope and diabetic hypoglycaemia can all cause episodes that look very like manifestations of epilepsy. Taken together, they are at least ten times commoner than epilepsy.

These children need very careful observation and diagnosis; their recognition and management are described in Stephenson's (1990) monograph *Fits and Faints*, which is studded with case histories and helpful advice; Chapter 14 describes 21 types of episode 'whose mechanisms are not clearly epileptic or anoxic, nor sufficiently peculiar to find a place in the chapter on psychic seizures.'

PATTERNS OF EPILEPSY DIFFER AS CHILDREN AGE

Neonatal seizures

Seizures are more likely to occur in the perinatal period than at any later stage in life. This subject is comprehensively covered in the textbooks by O'Donohoe (1994), Levene et al (1988), Murphy and Dehkarghani (1993) and Rust and Volpe (1994). Neonatal seizures may be the first sign of a nervous system disorder. In the premature infant fits can be difficult to differentiate from their normal jerky movement pattern. The clue that seizures are occurring tends to be localized jerky movements often involving the eyes; these abnormal movements may be missed by the inexperienced. It is essential to make immediate investigations so that appropriate treatment can be given without delay.

Possible causes include:

1. *Biochemical deficiency*: low blood sugar level; vitamin B_6 dependency, biotin deficiency, aminoacidopathy and organic acidopathy. Deficiency of calcium causes tetanic spasms which are not strictly seizures; these episodes may not respond until magnesium levels are normalized as well.

2. *Congenital*: structural malformation of the brain and ventricles that may or may not be associated with external abnormality. The following are especially associated with neonatal seizures: chromosomal abnormality of many types, neurofibromatosis, Sturge–Weber syndrome, tuberose sclerosis, congenital intracranial abnormality. *Smith's Recognizable Human Malformations* (Jones, 1992) lists 54 syndromes, mainly very rare, that are associated with seizures; even this is not fully inclusive. More are described by O'Donohoe in Chapter 2 of this volume.

   Few, however, can hope to be able to remember the clinical details of the rarer syndromes and need help from a clinical geneticist with access to a computer database of syndromes. It is particularly important that post-mortem examinations in undiagnosed cases are performed by paediatric pathologists and, if a diagnosis does not emerge, appropriate tissue specimens are stored in the expectation that future advances will lead to the diagnosis and eventually to informed genetic counselling.

3. *Infectious*: prenatal virus infection and early postnatal septicaemia with Gram-negative bacteria.

4. *Intrapartum trauma* leading to focal vascular ischaemia giving rise to focal seizures and hypotonia associated with intraventricular haemorrhage.

5. *Toxic*: hyperbilirubinaemia; bacterial toxic shock from enteric bacterial infection.

6. *Maternal drug effects*: withdrawal of opiates and barbiturates; accidental injection of lignocaine to the fetus.

7. *Benign and unexplained*: occasional infants develop transitory seizures, particularly around the fifth day; some are entirely benign instances of neonatal sleep myoclonus; the occasional awake infant manifests seizure-like episodes during gastro-oesophageal reflux. These are diagnoses of exclusion. Metabolic (Surtees and Leonard, 1994) and infectious causes must not be overlooked.

Post-neonatal and later in the first year

After the perinatal period new cases of seizures become less frequent (see Chapter 2). The National Childhood Encephalopathy Study (Alderslade et al, 1981) found that serious neurological illness in infancy was most likely to present at 8 months, often with seizures as the first sign. It is not known why the brain is relatively less seizure-prone in the earlier months. The study revealed a very wide range of diagnoses; in many cases the underlying cause could not be demonstrated. Among these infantile spasms is a particularly important condition; epidemiological studies suggest they affect between 1 in 3000 and 1 in 10 000 children, mainly in the age group of 6–12 months. Much more needs to be learnt about their nature and causation. They are not a heterogeneous disorder; careful examination can reveal a cause in up to 70% of cases (Bellman, 1983; Cowan and Hudson, 1991). Unresolved questions include:

1. Why is this condition virtually unique to this age group?
2. Why may one of identical twins develop spasms but not the other? Spasms are often missed until seen by a doctor who recognizes the condition; they can be readily dismissed as colic or just parental fussiness unless witnessed.
3. Is the administration of early intensive treatment with steroids truly beneficial or is early response merely an indicator of benign underlying disease?
4. What is their relation to Lennox–Gastaut syndrome (see Chapter 2; and Dulac and N'Guyen, 1993). This form of myoclonic epilepsy usually presents with both retardation and tonic and atonic seizures with a characteristic EEG with interictal spikes. Some, but not all, initially present with infantile spasms.

FEBRILE CONVULSIONS

Febrile convulsions are discussed in detail by Camfield and Camfield in Chapter 6. About 3% of children in temperate regions have had one or more febrile convulsion. Febrile convulsions pose many challenging unanswered questions including:

- Why do they occur?
- When should lumbar puncture be performed?
- Do febrile convulsions cause any lasting harm?
- If later, non-febrile epilepsy occurs, was it caused by the febrile convulsions?
- What is the role of inheritance?
- Why are febrile convulsions mainly confined to children in the age range of 6 months to 5 years?
- Is it worth giving prophylactic anticonvulsants?

NON-FEBRILE EPILEPSY: THE SIZE OF THE PROBLEM

There are inherent difficulties in determining both the prevalence and incidence of epilepsies in childhood (Cowan et al, 1989). These include: the possibility of a concealed diagnosis; an incorrect diagnosis; the definition of cure (does seizure suppression by drugs equal cure?); and whether an abnormal EEG or other investigative findings should be taken as diagnostic? This difficulty applies particularly in rare circumstances such as the Landau–Kleffner syndrome (see Chapter 2; Paquier et al, 1992), which involves loss of speech associated with a characteristic EEG, where there may be no clinical seizures. Should a disorder where the EEG is abnormal yet there are no clinical seizures be regarded as a form of epilepsy?

Studies based on hospital patients give biased information: findings depend on the hospital's catchment population; the higher the prestige of the hospital the greater the selection bias because some patients, particularly the wealthy, will travel long distances to be seen. Conversely, a hospital with a poor reputation may have a bias towards referral of milder cases and poorer patients. To overcome selection bias it is best to study patients directly from the local population. Some people, however, are unsure whether they have epilepsy or not; some will not reply to questionnaires; people move and records are lost.

The need for data

Data on populations with epilepsy are needed for reasons that include:

- *Causation*: a search is needed for clues regarding aetiology. To what extent do inherited, congenital, birth-related, postnatal accident and illness, and environmental factors have a bearing on causation? It is possible to ascertain whether an environmental factor is operating only if past data are available from the same and comparable populations. These data must be collected in a uniform manner using the same case definitions throughout.
- *Health service, social welfare, educational and employment provision.*

Is the epilepsy still active; in what proportion can epilepsy be regarded as 'cured'?

Two epidemiological dimensions need to be considered:

1. *Incidence*: the number of new cases that occurred in a defined population and period, usually 1 year, expressed as the rate per 1000 within a defined age span. This can be calculated from a cross-sectional study in which an attempt is made to study a defined, preferably entire, population by a census taken, if possible, on a specific day or in as short a time as possible.
2. *Prevalence*: the number of people in a community who can be regarded as having a tendency to epilepsy per 1000 of a defined age span. This rate on its own may not be very helpful; we may need to know how many actually had a fit in a defined time span (e.g. the 12 months preceding a particular day) so that the *active epilepsy rate* can be calculated. It is necessary to decide whether fits themselves should be the sole reason for inclusion; some studies retain those who are taking antiepilepsy drugs

yet are fit-free, or those in whom the EEG remains abnormal although there are no clinically recorded seizures. All too readily the study may reveal more about the prescribing habits of doctors than the prevalence of epilepsy *per se*. It is also possible to calculate the *cumulative prevalence*, which includes all who ever had a diagnosis of epilepsy. This requires a longitudinal study where the same population is followed over a period of time. These are much more labour intensive than cross-sectional studies, and may be difficult to interpret on account of population movements unless an entire 'captive' population is available.

Sources of epidemiological data

These are listed and discussed by Hauser et al (1991), Hauser and Annegers (1993), and Sander and Shorvon (1987), Shorvon (1990) and Sillanpåå (1992).

Cross-sectional studies

Islands form a good basis for epilepsy studies: Gudmundsson (1966) made a cross-sectional study of the whole population of Iceland, which has central-ized medical records, and undertook personal interviews 'in the freezing factories and fields'. Joënsen (1986) studied Faeroe islanders 20 years later. Rutter et al (1970) in the Isle of Wight (UK) studied epilepsy as part of an in-depth neuropsychiatric study of schoolchildren.

Longitudinal studies

The longest running study comes from Rochester County in the USA where people of all ages with epilepsy have been studied continuously since the 1930s and reported in a series of papers, of which a recent representative is that of Hauser and colleagues (1991).

In the USA, 50 000 babies born in a series of teaching hospitals were followed for their first 7 years by Nelson and Ellenberg (1976) as part of the Collaborative Perinatal Project and form the basis of a study into the prognosis of children with febrile convulsions. The only longitudinal studies that covered entire countries have been undertaken in the UK. They were based on perinatal studies that included virtually all births in single weeks in March or April 1946 (Cooper, 1965), 1958 (Ross et al, 1980) and 1970 (Verity et al, 1992). Studies were made of those who subsequently developed seizures, and the authors also throw light on the size and nature of populations with non-epileptic seizures, febrile convulsions and non-febrile epilepsy. The strength of these studies lies in the availability of massive numbers of control or reference cases, making it possible to look in depth at perinatal, developmental, illness, educational, behavioural and social factors. The 1946 study was based on a sample of 5000 survivors, while the 1958- and 1970-based studies included the entire original cohort, numbering 17 000 and 14 000 respectively, who were followed up through their school years and beyond into adult life. Lists of those with a history of episodes of altered consciousness were compiled with the help of treating physicians to determine whether the children had epilepsy and, if so, its nature, treatment and prognosis, social factors and educational achievement at school and employment obtained after leaving school. These studies are continuing and promise to give the most complete picture to date of epilepsy in a nation. Findings from the 1958 and 1970 studies have been summarized by Verity and Ross (1985). They include:

- At age 11 years, 4 per 1000 children were accepted as having a verified diagnosis of epilepsy, of whom about half had not had a fit in the previous 2 years.
- Two thirds were in mainstream education and one third in special education; most of the latter were multiply handicapped with a wide variety of associated conditions that were often more of a disability than the epilepsy per se, which was rarely the sole reason for special education.
- Children with epilepsy came from all social classes; there was a small excess of males.

Despite the 12 years between the studies, they gave very similar findings and suggest that there were no major changes in prevalence during this time period.

ARE THE EPILEPSIES PREVENTABLE DISORDERS?

Unfortunately, there do not appear to be any large-scale cohort studies of children with epilepsy in progress based on a current well-investigated population that could shed new light on the aetiology of the epilepsies. A source of such information is badly needed to determine which cases of epilepsy could be prevented, and the influence of new methods of investigation and treatment. We have to fall back on the now ageing information on aetiology gathered from the British longitudinal studies which were carried out before the current generation of investigations became available. In the 1958-based cohort, Ross et al (1980) found a possible cause for epilepsy in 25% of the 64 11-year-old children studied; about half of these cases could have been prevented given current knowledge or better luck. Even then, birth trauma (apart from maternal bleeding before 28 weeks) did not play a significant role; three were associated with syndromes that can now be diagnosed antenatally and decisions made about abortion. Trauma, both accidental and probably non-accidental, caused two cases, and there were four cases resulting from meningitis, which should eventually become preventable through immunization.

Pertussis, measles (particularly subacute sclerosing panencephalitis) and mumps related epilepsies have long been preventable through immunization. We need to know the impact of the survival of the formerly previable premature infants who are now being saved. Previously unrecognizable syndromes explain a few cases, usually associated with severe systemic abnormality such as Rett syndrome.

In a study of 100 consecutive local cases seen at a district hospital epilepsy clinic in London, no children born and brought up in the UK were regarded as having a potentially preventable epilepsy, although there were a number who acquired their epilepsy overseas in a developing country (Ross and Bommen, 1983).

PITFALLS IN ASSIGNING EPILEPSY DIAGNOSES

Up to 30 years ago childhood epilepsies after the first year were largely split into (i) 'grand mal' where there was generalized tonic–clonic spasms, often preceded by an aura and postictal sleep; (ii) much briefer petit mal episodes (the term petit mal is perhaps the most misused in epileptology—O'Donohoe, 1994); and (iii) psychomotor, which grouped together a host of ill-defined epilepsies associated with behavioural aspects. This inexact terminology was on a par with practice elsewhere in paediatrics; infants with serious and inoperable cardiac disorder were then referred to as having 'morbus cordis' and as being 'blue babies'.

The understanding of children's epilepsies has gone through a similar evolutionary process. The old nomenclature has been replaced by the concept of *epilepsy syndromes*, which are discussed in depth by O'Donohoe in Chapter 2 and by Roger et al (1992). The clinical features of these syndromes, however, can change as the child matures, and it is easy to make mistakes leading to the prescription of unsuitable therapy and the wrong prognosis (Gordon and Aird, 1991).

Incorrect diagnosis

The following types of epilepsy are often muddled up.

Absence attacks

Childhood absence epilepsy. This diagnosis should be made only in those few children, more girls than boys, who have brief episodes of unconsciousness **without** an aura, falling or urination, or postictal sleep; the only signs are fluttering of the eyelids and twitching of the nares. The EEG shows a diagnostic 3-Hz spike and wave (dart and dome) pattern. This type of epilepsy still tends to be overdiagnosed, the old name (petit mal) had a reassuring ring to it and was often wrongly used to describe quite different forms of epilepsy, especially myoclonic absences.

Myoclonic absences. These are more common in boys; the pattern of attack is more complex and involves bilateral clonic jerking. This type of epilepsy tends to be much more resistant to standard therapy. There is a tendency to intellectual deterioration; a concurrent EEG and polygraphic record of muscular movements helps to clinch the diagnosis.

Complex partial epilepsies

The temporal lobe and within it the hippocampal gyrus and surrounding structures, especially the amygdala, are the key to understanding the *complex partial epilepsies* that comprise 10–24% of cases of epilepsy in schoolchildren (Bruton, 1988). Whether the majority are due to congenital abnormality or are secondary to later cerebral ischaemia remains the focus of a long-running debate. Once this matter is settled we will be much nearer to understanding the essential nature of the partial epilepsies. Recognition and accurate diagnosis is essential so that all treatment options, including surgery, can be fully explored. This requires a team including neurophysiologist, neuroradiologist and paediatrician able to gain the confidence of the child, parents and teachers.

Juvenile myoclonic epilepsy (JME)

This type of epilepsy is also known as the Janz syndrome. This rare epilepsy has a good prognosis; there is myoclonic limb jerking, especially of the upper arms on waking. The EEG shows polyspikes but also myoclonus if appropriate leads are studied. There is a genetic abnormality on chromosome 6, discussed by Hodgson and Verity in Chapter 3. Sodium valproate is usually effective but has to be taken on a long-term basis.

Progressive myoclonic epilepsy (PME)

This term sounds very similar to JME, readily causing confusion, but is a very different kettle of fish. The occurrence of PME suggests an evolving severe neurodegenerative disorder, such as juvenile Gaucher, sialidosis, Ramsay Hunt syndrome or Lafora body disorder. PME tends to present with occasional non-specific seizures that may initially appear to be an attention-seeking device. Their progressive nature sooner or later leads the child to a neurological clinic. Recognition is important so that the parents can at least be given a rational understanding of the problem, but response to antiepileptic drug treatment is poor.

Benign partial epilepsy of childhood with focal centrotemporal spikes (benign nocturnal focal Rolandic epilepsy)

These attacks usually, but not invariably, occur during sleep. The prognosis is very good, males predominate, there are usually no abnormal neurological signs and intelligence is normal. Although it has been reported from Scandinavia (Heijbel et al, 1975) that this type of epilepsy accounts for 16% of cases of epilepsy in teenagers, this high proportion has not been reported elsewhere. It is extremely difficult to know whether clinical surveys really pick up all these cases and the extent to which similar EEG changes are found in a clinically fit-free population.

Classifiable, unclassified and unclassifiable epilepsy

More and more forms of epilepsy are being described. Some such as frontal (Stores et al, 1991; Scheffer et al, 1994) or occipital (Panayiotopoulos, 1993) relate to the area of maximal EEG abnormality; others to proposed causes such as reading frightening literature—one patient attributed his fits to the book *Jaws*, although more innocuous literature can have the same effect.

INTERNATIONAL CLASSIFICATION

It becomes clear that defining epilepsy by either presumed aetiology, EEG changes or area of brain affected is illogical and leads to confusion. For this reason a classification scheme akin to that devised by Linnaeus in connection with botany over 200 years ago was long needed. After several earlier attempts an International Classification of the Epilepsies (Commission on Classification, 1989) has been introduced; the rationale for it is discussed in detail in Chapter 2. Please use this classification. If you still want to use the old terms, put them in parentheses.

The international classification is based on aetiology, not seizure type, and focuses thought on prevention. A seizure disorder can be primary, secondary or unclassified, partial or generalized.

To use the international classification it is necessary to make a diagnosis of the types of epilepsy. The basis for this should be obvious, but elementary mistakes are commonly made because the old rules are not followed. They are described below.

History and examination

A full history should be supplied by someone who has actually witnessed the attacks as well as by the parents who may not have seen them. If at all possible a videotape of the attacks is extremely valuable (increasingly, parents are able to supply this).

A full examination of the eventually undressed child should be performed, with attention to development, growth in weight, height and occipitofrontal circumference. Fundi should be checked and blood pressure taken. The skin may yield clues of tuberose sclerosis, neurofibromatoma and port wine stains.

EEG

When correctly performed, the EEG gives a useful insight into cerebral electrical behaviour but must not be allowed to take the place of clinical diagnosis; a normal EEG does not rule out a diagnosis of epilepsy. There is considerable risk of varying opinions being given on the same record. The standard record lasts about 20 min and may need to be supplemented by sleep recordings or 24-h portable monitoring. Neurophysiologists are experienced clinicians; they can give the fullest interpretation of the EEG only if they are given full clinical details and are invited to become involved in clinical management. Neurophysiology is discussed in detail by Binnie in Chapter 8.

Brain scanning

The advent of computed tomography (CT) in the early 1970s promised to revolutionize diagnosis in epilepsy, and there were those who prophesied the end of the EEG. They have long been proved wrong. The majority of children with normal intelligence and epilepsy have normal CT scan appearances. CT is particularly useful for demonstrating the shape of ventricles, presence of the corpus callosum, vascular anomalies and intracranial calcification. CT is being rapidly superseded by magnetic resonance imaging (MRI), which gives no irradiation and much enhanced detailing, perhaps revealing a small glioma not apparent on the CT scan. As with all investigations, it is vital that the record is undertaken and read by those who are appropriately experienced and that the correct views are taken. Intracranial calcification is poorly shown on MRI. In preoperative assessment, further techniques including brain mapping are useful.

ANTIEPILEPSY DRUGS

Many parents dislike the thought of their child having long-term medication. Both over and under medication can cause great harm. Decisions must not be left to the inexperienced. There are two schools of thought about starting drug therapy: (i) the kindling theory that each fit paves the way to the next and that prognosis is better if drug treatment is started early in full fit-suppressing dosage; and (ii) the view that antiepilepsy drugs do no more than suppress seizure occurrence and do nothing to affect underlying brain pathology. Adherents to the latter view will point out that all anticonvulsants have side-effects and recall rodent-based experiments showing that chronically administered drugs result in underdevelopment of the growing brain (Iivanainen, 1983).

Drugs are not the only factor in treatment. In Chapter 5 Schwartz discusses the role of diet and surgery, and assesses unorthodox treatment. Treatment decisions are discussed by Shinnar (1994).

Compliance with drugs, diet and other advice is often poor (Buchanan, 1993). The truth about drug compliance may be revealed by blood levels. The dose needed tends to vary between children during rapid growth and may need frequent adjustment. The advent of puberty *per se* does not usually herald a significant change in the severity of seizures, although absence seizures usually cease by this age. A small minority of cases of epilepsy are very resistant to treatment (Livingston, 1991). The drug management of children with epilepsy hs been reviewed by Wallace (1992):

1. The side-effects of antiepilepsy drugs can be difficult to spot, particularly in a child who has been taking them for a long time.
2. Clumsiness, depression and poor school performance may be due to brain abnormality, drug side-effects or a low-grade manifestation of epilepsy. Many children became much livelier when the drug is changed to a more appropriate one, or discontinued (Matthew et al, 1982; Meador et al, 1990).

3. It is best to choose an antiepilepsy drug from a limited number of drugs whose nature one knows well.
4. Some children have atypical drug intolerance not described in medical literature. It is important to note parental observations and be prepared to act on them.
5. In general, monotherapy is the correct policy; giving more than one anticonvulsant drug at a time may lead to unexpected drug interactions.

How long to keep a child on anticonvulsants after the last fit

Gowers in 1881, in relation to bromides, suggested that therapy should be continued for 2–3 years after the last fit, but no hard evidence accrued until the British Medical Research Council's Antiepileptic Drug Withdrawal Group reported in 1991. There is no point in continuing a drug if it is not showing clear benefit. There are no absolute rules that apply to all children; understanding the nature and thus the expected prognosis of the different epilepsy syndromes is a great help, and guidelines are beginning to emerge.

Available anticonvulsants

After a 20-year interval following the introduction of sodium valproate and carbamazepine, a host of new anticonvulsants is under intensive investigation and a number have been launched on to some, but not all, international markets; the licences usually apply only to adults but some can be prescribed for children on a named-patient basis only. Children's doctors would be wise not to rush into their use and to insist on seeing the results of collaborative trials before changing their prescribing habits. The young child often reacts differently to drugs from adults. It is, however, likely that some of these drugs will become important in paediatric practice.

Currently available antiepilepsy drugs were introduced in three main time spans: (1) 1910–1960—phenobarbitone, phenytoin/dilantin, ethosuximide, primidone; (2) 1960–1970—carbamazepine, sodium valproate, clonazepam, diazepam, nitrazepam; and (3) 1990 onwards—gabapentin, lamotrigine, vigabatrin, feldamate, oxycarbamazepine.

New drugs tend to be licensed initially for prescription to children with epilepsy refractory to other drugs and initial experience is gained with their use in combination. There are great difficulties in developing the 'perfect' drug that not only controls seizures but also has the fewest possible side-effects; some drugs have powerful effects on mood and behaviour that are very difficult to quantify in the developing child.

The choice of anticonvulsant is rarely straightforward. Some types of epilepsy are unresponsive to certain drugs; some children have forms of epilepsy that cannot be put into a clear-cut category. There is much individual variation in dose–response and side-effects. In the newborn, there is still little firm evidence about the toxicity of the newer drugs; diazepam as a rapidly acting short-life measure and phenobarbitone with its long half-life remain the drugs of choice.

PROGNOSIS OF EPILEPSY

Much depends on whether the child is one of the third with multiple handicap. These children often have a mental disability and this, rather than the fits, may be the greatest problem. Two thirds go to normal schools and most do well, although they are often subject to needless restrictions, anxiety and overprotection leading to a 'chip on shoulder' and under-achievement. The psychosocial problems of those with chronic epilepsy is discussed by Hoare and Kerley (1991) and academic underachievement by Mitchell et al (1991).

TRUTHFUL EXPLANATION TO CHILD AND PARENT

Both child and parent need to understand as much as possible about epilepsy to counteract mistruths. The word epilepsy should not be hidden, and must be used where appropriate.

ROLE OF PROFESSIONAL AND VOLUNTARY SOCIETIES FOR EPILEPSY

Patient-oriented societies exist in all developed and in many developing countries. They depend on clinicians for professional advice and raise money for research. There is an obligation on paediatricians to tell parents about the existence of these voluntary societies and to urge them to take advantage of the advice and support that they can give. The International League against Epilepsy, a federation of local national chapters, organizes both local and international conferences and promotes co-operation in the spread of information and the development of internationally recognized classification schemes. Reports of their biannual conferences are published by Raven Press, New York.

PROVISION OF CARE: A POINT FOR DISCUSSION

Who should provide medical care for the child with epilepsy? Is there a case for specialist 'epileptologist's' medical and nursing, or should the service continue as at present with the bulk of the work done by generalists of whom a few take a special personal interest in epilepsy? Most developed countries have very few special epilepsy centres, usually built around a group of individuals who have built up indepth knowledge of epilepsy in childhood; these organizations naturally wax and wane in influence, and their future generally depends more on personal initiatives than long-term planning.

So far, no controlled studies have been undertaken to determine whether children who attend special centres make better progress than those who attend local general clinics, although it is apparent elsewhere in children's medicine (e.g. cystic fibrosis, diabetes, leukaemia) that those who attend research-based regional centres make the best progress.

There is much anecdotal evidence that the overall quality of management of epilepsy in children and young people with epilepsy is very variable, particularly among those with other disabilities. Unpublished findings from the subjects of the National Child Development Study born in 1958 show that those with epilepsy who were in mainstream education with epilepsy at the age of 11 years have a high chance of loosing their fits, and in some cases of forgetting that they ever had epilepsy; those with multiple problems, mainly educational handicap plus epilepsy, had a much poorer prognosis. Thomas et al (1989), in a study of 104 young British handicapped adults of whom one third (31) had a diagnosis of epilepsy, concluded: 'Polypharmacy was very common, and many young people were taking tranquillisers, although the reason for the initial prescription was often difficult to ascertain. Several caretakers admitted that they failed to renew prescriptions in time . . . some remarked that it seemed to make little difference to the level or frequency of epileptic fits whether anticonvulsive drugs were taken or not.'

In the past 30 years three UK government enquiries into services for people with epilepsy have reached similar conclusions—that epilepsy services should be upgraded and special regional centres created in order to service peripheral clinics and thus raise standards throughout the country. These reports have been debated in parliament, the conclusions agreed, but no special finance earmarked; thus few changes have occurred (Morrow, 1993).

In the UK an 'epilepsy special needs' group has been set up to write a document outlining the needs for epilepsy services in the population as a basis for health-purchasing authorities to commission services from providing organizations (Brown et al, 1993). Chadwick and colleagues (1993) have produced an updated review of the quality of life and care in epilepsy.

BUILDING A LIBRARY ON EPILEPSY IN CHILDREN

Aicardi J (1993) *Epilepsy in Children*, 2nd edn. New York: Raven Press.
Brett E (1992) *Paediatric Neurology*, 2nd edn. Edinburgh: Churchill Livingstone.
Engel J (ed.) (1994) *Surgical Treatment of the Epilepsies*, 2nd edn. New York: Raven Press.
Levene MI, Bennett MJ & Punt J (eds) (1988) *Fetal and Neonatal Neurology and Neurosurgery*. Edinburgh: Churchill Livingstone.
Murphy JV & Dehkarghani (eds) (1993) *Handbook of Pediatric Epilepsy*. New York: Dekker.
Nelson K and Ellenberg JH (1981) *Febrile Seizures*. New York: Raven Press.
O'Donohoe NV (1994) *Epilepsies of Childhood*, 3rd edn. Oxford: Butterworth–Heinemann.
Roger J et al (eds) (1992) *Epileptic Syndromes in Infancy, Childhood and Adolescence*. Paris: John Libbey.
Schwartzkroin PA (ed.) (1993) *Epilepsy. Models, Mechanisms and Concepts*. Cambridge: Cambridge University Press.
Stephenson JB (1990) *Fits and Faints*. Oxford: MacKeith Press.
Volpe JJ (1987) *Neurology of the Newborn*, 2nd edn. Philadelphia: Saunders.

PAEDIATRIC CHAPTERS IN A BOOK ON EPILEPSY

Hauser WA & Annegers JF (1993) Epidemiology of epilepsy. In Laidlaw J, Richens A & Chadwick D (eds) *Textbook of Epilepsy*, 4th edn, pp 23–45. Edinburgh: Churchill Livingstone.
Wallace SJ (1993) Seizures in children. In Laidlaw J, Richens A & Chadwick D (eds) *Textbook of Epilepsy*, 4th edn, pp 77–164. Edinburgh: Churchill Livingstone.

SERIAL VOLUMES

Pedley TA & Meldrum B (eds) *Recent Advances in Epilepsy*, vols 1–5. Edinburgh: Churchill Livingstone.

BOOKS FOR PARENTS (AND CHILDREN'S DOCTORS)

Chadwick D & Usiskin S (1987) *Living with Epilepsy*. London: Macdonald-Optima.
Freeman JM, Vining EPG & Pillas DJ (1990) *Seizures and Epilepsy in Childhood: A Guide for Parents*. Baltimore: Johns Hopkins Press.

HISTORICAL SOURCES

Lennox WG & Lennox MA (1960) *Epilepsy and Related Disorders*. Boston: Little, Brown & Company.
Tempkin O (1971) *The Falling Sickness*, 2nd edn. Baltimore: Johns Hopkins Press.

REFERENCES IN TEXT

Alderslade R, Bellman MH, Rawson NSB et al (1981) The National Childhood Encephalopathy Study. Chapters v–viii, pp 79–169. In *Whooping Cough*. London: HMSO.
Bellman H (1983) Infantile spasms. In Pedley TA & Meldrum BS (eds) *Recent Advances in Epilepsy*, vol. 1, pp 113–138. Edinburgh: Churchill Livingstone.
Berg AT & Shinner S (1991) The risk of seizure recurrence following a first unprovoked seizure. A quantitative review. *Neurology* 41: 965–972.
Betts T (1990) Pseudoseizures: seizures that are not epilepsy. *Lancet* 336: 163–164.
Brown S, Betts T, Chadwick D et al (1993) An epilepsy needs document. *Seizure* 2: 91–103.
Bruton CJ (1988) *The Neuropathology of Temporal Lobe Epilepsy*. Oxford: Oxford University Press.
Buchanan N (1993) Noncompliance with medication amongst persons attending a tertiary referral epilepsy clinic: implications, management and outcome. *Seizure* 2: 79–82.
Buchanan N & Snars J (1993) Pseudoseizures (nonepileptic attack disorder)—clinical management and outcome in 50 patients. *Seizure* 2: 141–146.
Chadwick DW, Baker GA & Jacoby A (eds) (1993) *Quality of Life and the Quality of Care in Epilepsy: Update 1993*. London: Royal Society of Medicine.
Commission on Classification and Terminology of the International League Against Epilepsy (1989) Proposal for revised classification of epilepsies and epileptic syndromes. *Epilepsia* 30: 389–399.
Cooper JE (1965) Epilepsy in a longitudinal survey of 5000 children. *British Medical Journal* 1: 1020–1022.
Cowan LD & Hudson LS (1991) The epidemiology and natural history of infantile spasms. *Journal of Child Neurology* 6: 355–364.

Cowan LD, Leviton A, Bodensteiner JB & Doherty L (1989) Problems in estimating the prevalence of epilepsy in children: the yield from different sources of information. *Paediatric and Perinatal Epidemiology* **3:** 386–401.

Dulac O & N'Guyen T (1993) The Lennox–Gastaut syndrome. *Epilepsia* **34 (supplement 7):** S7–S17.

Gordon N & Aird RB (1991) Idiopathic childhood epilepsies, a system disorder: its diagnosis and differentiation. *Developmental Medicine and Child Neurology* **33:** 744–748.

Gowers W (1881) *Epilepsy and Other Chronic Diseases*, pp 301. London: Churchill.

Gudmundsson G (1966) Epilepsy in Iceland: a clinical and epidemiological investigation. *Acta Neurologica Scandinavica. Supplementum* **25(43):** 1–124.

Hart YM, Sander JWAS, Johnson AL & Shorvon SD (1990) National general practice study of epilepsy: recurrence after a first seizure. *Lancet* **336:** 1271–1274.

Hauser WA, Annegers JF & Kurland LT (1991) Prevalence of epilepsy in Rochester, Minnesota: 1940–1980. *Epilepsia* **27(32):** 429–454.

Heijbel J, Bloom S & Bergfors PG (1975) Benign epilepsy of children with centrotemporal EEG foci: a study the incidence rate in outpatient care. *Epilepsia* **16:** 657–664.

Hoare P & Kerley S (1991) Psychosocial adjustment of children with chronic epilepsy and their families. *Developmental Medicine and Child Neurology* **33:** 201–215.

Iivanainen MV (1983) Effects of antiepileptic drugs on maturation of the human body. In Morselli PK, Pippenger CE & Penry JK (eds) *Antiepileptic Drug Therapy in Pediatrics*, pp 65–73. New York: Raven Press.

Joënsen P (1986) Prevalence, incidence and classification of epilepsy in Faroes. *Acta Neurologica Scandinavica* **74:** 150–155.

Jones KL (1992) Smith's *Recognizable Patterns of Human Malformation*. 4th edition. pp 708–709. Philadelphia: WB Saunders.

Livingston JH (1991) Management of intractable epilepsy. *Archives of Disease in Childhood* **66:** 1454–1456.

Matthew WS, Barabas G & Ferrari M (1982) Emotional concomitants of childhood epilepsy. *Epilepsia* **23:** 671–681.

Meador KJ, Loring DW, Huh K et al (1990) Comparative cognitive effects of anticonvulsants. *Neurology* **40:** 391–394.

Meadow R (1991) Neurological and developmental variants of Munchausen syndrome by proxy. *Journal of Developmental Medicine and Child Neurology* **33:** 270–272.

Medical Research Council Antiepileptic Drug Withdrawal Group (1991) *Lancet* **337:** 1175–1180.

Metrick MF, Ritter FJ, Gates JR et al (1991) Nonepileptic events in childhood epilepsy. *Epilepsia* **32:** 322–328.

Mitchell WG, Chavez JM, Lee H et al (1991) Academic underachievement in children with epilepsy. *Journal of Child Neurology* **6:** 65–72.

Morrow JI (1993) Specialized epilepsy clinics. *Seizure* **2:** 267–268.

Nelson KB & Ellenberg JH (1976) Predictors of epilepsy in children who have experienced febrile seizures. *New England Journal of Medicine* **259:** 1029–1033.

Panayiotopoulos CP (1993) Benign childhood epilepsy with occipital paroxysms. In Andermann F, Beaumanoir A, Mira L et al (eds) *Occipital Seizures and Epilepsies in Children*, Chapter 28, pp 151–164. London: John Libbey.

Paquier PF, van Dongen HR & Loonen CB (1992) The Landau–Kleffner syndrome or acquired aphasia with convulsive disorder: long term follow up of six children and a review of the literature. *Archives of Neurology* **49:** 354–359.

Reynolds EH (1988) Historical aspects. In Trimble MR & Reynolds EH (eds) *Epilepsy, Behaviour and Cognitive Function*, pp 3–8. Chichester: John Wiley.

Ross EM & Bommen M (1983) An epilepsy clinic for children: analysis of a year's work. *Journal of Clinical Practice (supplement)* 105–108.

Ross EM, Peckham CS, West PB & Butler NR (1980) Epilepsy in childhood: findings from the National Child Development Study. *British Medical Journal* **i:** 207–210.

Rust RS & Volpe JJ (1994) Neonatal seizures. In Dodson WE & Pellock JM (eds) *Pediatric Epilepsy: Diagnosis and Therapy*, New York: Demos.

Rutter M, Graham P & Yule W (1970) A neuropsychiatric study in childhood. In *Clinics in Developmental Medicine*, nos35/36, Part 3, pp 99–162. London: Spastics International Medical Publications/Heinemann.

Sander JWAS & Shorvon SD (1987) Incidence and prevalence studies in epilepsy and their methodological problems: a review. *Journal of Neurology, Neurosurgery and Psychiatry* **50:** 829–839.

Scheffer IE, Bhatia KP, Lopes-Cendes I et al (1994) Autosomal dominant frontal epilepsy misdiagnosed as sleep disorder. *Lancet* **343:** 515–517.

Shinnar S (1994) Treatment decisions in childhood seizures. In Dodson WE & Pellock JM (eds) *Pediatric Epilepsy: Diagnosis and Therapy*. New York: Demos.

Shorvon SD (1990) Epidemiology, classification, natural history of epilepsy. *Lancet* **336:** 93–96.

Sillanpää M (1992) Epilepsy in children: prevalence, disability and handicap. *Epilepsia* **33:** 444–449.

Stores G, Zaiwalla Z & Bergel N (1991) Frontal lobe complex partial seizures in children: a form of epilepsy at particular risk of misdiagnosis. *Developmental Medicine and Child Neurology* **33:** 998–1009.

Surtees RAH & Leonard JV (1994) Metabolic encephalopathy in inborn errors of metabolism. In Eyre JA (ed.) *Coma—Clinical Paediatrics Series*, pp 65–80. London: Baillière Tindall.

Thomas AP, Bax MCO & Smyth DPL (1989) In *The health and social needs of young adults with physical disabilities*, pp 55. Oxford: MacKeith Press/Blackwell.

Verity CM & Ross EM (1985) Longitudinal studies of children's epilepsy. In Ross E & Reynolds (eds) *Paediatric perspectives on epilepsy*, pp 133–140. Chichester: Wiley.

Verity CM, Ross EM & Golding J (1992) Epilepsy in the first ten years of life: findings of the child health and education study. *British Medical Journal* **307:** 857–861.

Wallace SJ (1992) Drug management of epilepsy. *Developmental Medicine and Child Neurology* **34:** 1018–1021.

2

Classification of epilepsies in infancy, childhood and adolescence

NIALL V. O'DONOHOE

Classifications are a means of conveying information. They should be relatively easy to use and reflect the needs of the user. Uniform classifications of any disease are necessary for its proper understanding, to promote better communication and facilitate the exchange of scientific information, and to study prognosis and decide on appropriate therapy. During the past two decades, the diagnosis and management of epilepsy have been enhanced by improved classification systems, by modern methods of neuroimaging and by the rational use of the established and more recently developed antiepileptic drugs (O'Donohoe, 1991).

The concept of the epilepsies, rather than epilepsy, is now generally recognized and accepted. Seizures, the clinical signs of the epilepsies, are perceived as the behavioural manifestations of a diverse group of underlying states of brain dysfunction rather than originating from a single cause (see discussion on clinical and genetic heterogeneity in Chapter 3). Because there is no single epilepsy, there cannot be a single cause or cure.

Epileptic seizures result from the sudden, excessive, electrical discharges of large aggregates of neurones, and their clinical components depend on the site of origin of the discharges and their mode of propagation in the brain. *Epileptogenesis* is a term that refers to the dynamic processes underlying the development of epilepsy. Epileptogenesis occurs when the functional balance between excitation and inhibition is disturbed in the brain and, in the rapidly changing brain of the infant and young child, this balance is constantly altering, influenced by maturational factors and by disease and modified by subcortical and interhemispheric events. For example, the substantia nigra, which has strong inhibitory effects through its γ-aminobutyric acid (GABA)ergic output, is considered to function inadequately in the immature organism (Moshé et al, 1987).

Traditional classifications of epilepsy were based on either aetiology or symptomatology. In those based on aetiology, the distinction between primary (or idiopathic) and secondary (or symptomatic) epilepsy was made, depending on whether an anatomically demonstrable brain lesion could be found. Classifications derived from symptomatology were seizure-oriented and differentiation was based on the clinical characteristics of the seizures. Hughlings Jackson (Taylor et al, 1931) first expressed the idea that a

Baillière's Clinical Paediatrics—
Vol. 2, No. 3, August 1994
ISBN 0–7020–1862–7

471

classification of epilepsy should take into account anatomical lesions, physiological disturbances of function and pathological processes. He was also the first to introduce the concept of generalized and partial seizures, and he recognized that partial seizures resulted from a focal disturbance in cerebral grey matter. Later, the advent and development of electro-encephalography (EEG) revealed the neurophysiological disturbances of function underlying epileptic seizures and, more recently, neuroimaging techniques have shown the multiple abnormalities of structure that may be associated with epilepsy (Holmes, 1989). Molecular genetic studies are now beginning to unravel the mysteries of the genetic predisposition in the so-called idiopathic or primary epilepsies (Leppert et al, 1989).

CLASSIFICATION OF SEIZURES

The modern era in seizure classification dates from 1969 when the Commission of the International League Against Epilepsy proposed a classification that is now regarded as a landmark (Gastaut, 1970). The development and diversification of objective methods of documenting seizures, including prolonged EEG recording and the use of videotape, have facilitated accurate descriptions of seizure types and their classification according to the dynamic process of clinical evolution of individual seizures. Synchronized videotape–EEG monitoring, using a split-screen technique, is now being used increasingly in many centres for the diagnosis and delineation of seizure types (American Academy of Neurology, 1989).

The most recent classification of epileptic seizures, an elaboration of the 1969 classification, was adopted by the Commission on Classification and Terminology of the International League Against Epilepsy (ILAE) in 1981 and is now widely accepted and used. Seizures are divided into generalized seizures, which may be convulsive or non-convulsive, and partial seizures, previously called focal seizures.

Generalized seizures are associated with bilateral cerebral hemisphere involvement, bilateral EEG discharges, bilateral clinical manifestations and loss of consciousness. They are subdivided into:

1. Absence seizures; atypical absence seizures
2. Myoclonic seizures
3. Clonic seizures
4. Tonic seizures
5. Tonic–clonic seizures
6. Atonic seizures

Partial seizures are those in which the initial clinical and EEG changes indicate activation of a system of neurones limited to part of one cerebral hemisphere. A partial seizure is classified primarily on the basis of whether consciousness is retained or impaired during the attack, impairment of consciousness being defined as a loss of awareness and/or responsiveness. Alterations of behaviour, called *automatisms*, may occur while consciousness is impaired. Partial seizures are subdivided into:

1. *Simple partial seizures*, during which there is no impairment of con-
    sciousness. These may present with motor, somatosensory, special
    sensory, autonomic or psychic symptoms, depending on which part of
    the brain is involved in the abnormal electrical events.
2. *Complex partial seizures*, during which consciousness is impaired; such
    alteration of consciousness may be the first clinical sign of the com-
    mencement of the attack. However, this type of seizure may be
    preceded by and evolve out of a simple partial seizure which then
    represents the *aura* preceding the complex partial seizure. Auras often
    consist of bizarre psychic, autonomic or special sensory symptoms
    (visceral and olfactory sensations, distortions of perception, visual and
    auditory hallucinations, sensations of fear or vertigo).
3. Either type of partial seizure may not terminate but instead progress
    into a *secondary generalized seizure* with complete loss of consciousness
    and generalized tonic–clonic movements.

Recognition of specific seizure patterns is of immediate and practical
importance for the clinician, and correct classification of seizures is essential
when choosing appropriate antiepileptic drug therapy. Nevertheless, for a
proper understanding of the nature of the childhood epilepsies, it is essential
to look beyond the presenting symptoms to try to determine the nature of
the underlying condition responsible for causing the seizures. The seizure
type simply represents the area of the nervous system involved by the
abnormal discharges. The underlying aetiological cause of the epilepsy has
implications for genetics, for higher cortical function and intelligence, for
the natural history of the disease, its response to medication and its
prognosis. Dreifuss (1990) has compared the individual seizure type to one
pigment with which the picture of the illness is painted. However, the whole
picture is composed of many pigments and their management is often
specific to a particular epilepsy.

CLASSIFICATIONS OF THE EPILEPSIES

Classifying the epilepsies, as distinct from classifying seizures, has always
presented problems, mainly because such a classification suggests a classification of diseases and, in fact, very few epileptic disease entities have been
defined (e.g. tuberous sclerosis). In recent years, there has been an increasing tendency to concentrate on the delineation of recognizable *epileptic
syndromes*, rather than attempting to devise a complete classification of the
epilepsies.

   In 1989, the Commission on Classification and Terminology of the
International League Against Epilepsy (ILAE) proposed an *International
Classification of Epilepsies and Epileptic Syndromes*. In this rather elaborate
classification, a division was made according to seizure type and EEG
findings into: (a) partial (or localization related); and (b) generalized; and
according to aetiology into: (a) idopathic (usually with an age-related
onset); and (b) symptomatic.

The term *cryptogenic* rather than idiopathic or primary was used for certain serious age-related syndromes (West's, Lennox–Gastaut), which are presumed to be symptomatic even though their precise cause remains to be discovered. The classification also allowed for anatomical differentiation, for example into frontal lobe, occipital or temporal lobe epilepsies.

EPILEPTIC SYNDROMES

As already emphasized, an epileptic seizure is an event, the symptom with which a neurological disorder presents. The condition of which the seizure is a symptom is the epilepsy or epileptic syndrome. During the past two decades, it has been possible to identify, during childhood and adolescence, a considerable number of epileptic syndromes, of which individual seizures are but one manifestation (Roger et al, 1992). Although the seizure may draw attention to the existence of a syndrome, the complete syndrome is composed of a cluster of signs and symptoms customarily occurring together. These include seizure type(s), family history, age of onset, natural history, interictal and ictal EEGs, neurological–psychological findings, response to antiepileptic drugs and aetiology.

In terms of the ILAE classification of epilepsies and epileptic syndromes, two main syndromic subgroups can be identified, namely idiopathic or primary and symptomatic or secondary syndromes. In *primary epileptic syndromes*, the seizures constitute the disease; no pathology can be identified. They are usually age-related, have a strong genetic component, respond well to medication or may not need medication, often remit spontaneously and may be characterized by highly specific clinical seizures. It is, however, important not to equate primary with benign in this context since some primary syndromes may cause life-long problems for the patient (e.g. juvenile myoclonic epilepsy).

In the *secondary epileptic syndromes*, the seizure is a symptom of an underlying neurological disorder and the medical history usually provides evidence of other patterns of brain dysfunction. They are often associated with underlying brain disease and with resulting neurodevelopmental abnormality. A positive family history is less likely, the response to medication is unpredictable and remission uncertain.

It should be remembered that similar seizures may occur in different primary and secondary epileptic syndromes and that some syndromes are characterized by multiple seizure types. Furthermore, syndromes vary in specificity from those that represent broad concepts to those that are highly specific, some having biochemical and chromosomal markers (Delgado-Escueta et al, 1989; Aicardi, 1992).

It must be admitted that there are inconsistencies when attempting to make clear-cut distinctions between primary and secondary epileptic syndromes. Some syndromes, such as West's syndrome and the Lennox–Gastaut syndrome, while usually symptomatic in their aetiology, nevertheless contain certain idiopathic and apparently primary variants—usually termed cryptogenic cases. These are without evidence of brain damage and usually have an unblemished neurodevelopmental record up to the onset of their seizures.

However, although the concept of epileptic syndromes does not embrace all types of convulsive disorder by any means, it has changed clinical attitudes to and management of these conditions. It probably has more practical application in the paediatric population than in the epileptic population at large. In a large population-based UK study, Manford et al (1992) could categorize only one third of their patients as having a specific ILAE syndrome. Recognizing the diagnostic difficulties, Berkovic and colleagues (1987) proposed an alternative *neurobiological approach* based on the evidence for a multifactorial origin of the generalized epilepsies in particular. In these, there is often a mixture of genetic and acquired factors and the patients demonstrate a spectrum of clinical and EEG features with often no clear distinction between primary and secondary types. This approach attempts to place the individual patient into a biological continuum that extends from the most genetically determined to the most obviously acquired type of epilepsy and uses clinical, neurophysiological, neuropsychological and radiological data to build a profile of the patient, an 'epileptic phenotype'. This method can be regarded as being complementary to and as extending the scope of the syndromic method of classification.

The categorization of the childhood epilepsies according to their *chronology* has a particular appeal for the practising paediatrician. During infancy, childhood and adolescence, the factors of age, growth and development are of particular importance in determining whether epilepsy develops or not. Age also dictates the type of syndrome that develops in some instances and influences the prognosis. Aicardi (1986) distinguishes four periods or epochs in the chronology of childhood epilepsy, as follows:

1. A neonatal period, extending to 3 months of age.
2. A period from 3 months to 4 years of age.
3. A period extending from 4 years to 9–10 years of age.
4. A period from 9–10 years onwards into adolescence.

This scheme is useful as a general diagnostic and prognostic framework. Using this method, and bearing in mind that many of the childhood epilepsies cannot be precisely categorized and that many of the recognized syndromes are rare, an account of the most important epilepsies and syndromes follows (O'Donohoe, 1992a). For a comprehensive account of the many different syndromes, the reader is referred to the monograph by Roger et al (1992).

Neonatal period to 3 months

During this period, seizures are frequently related to structural pathology and the prognosis is poor. Neonatal seizures are usually partial in type and difficult to recognize. Hypoxic–ischaemic encephalopathy, metabolic disorders, brain malformations, chromosomal abnormalities and narcotic withdrawal may be responsible. Tonic posturing and various motor automatisms, previously regarded as epileptic seizures, are now considered to be non-epileptic brain-stem release phenomena (Scher and Painter, 1989). Two epileptic syndromes have been defined. *Benign idiopathic neonatal convulsions* or 'fifth-day fits' present between 3 and 7 days in otherwise normal infants, without obvious aetiology. Frequent clonic multi-focal seizures occur which may be associated with apnoea or cyanosis. They recur for less than 48 h and then remit without sequelae (Pryor et al, 1981). *Benign familial neonatal convulsions* constitute a rare syndrome that is inherited in an autosomal dominant fashion, and linkage to chromosome 20 has been demonstrated (Leppert et al, 1989). Clonic or apnoeic seizures occur as early as 2–3 days or as late as 3 months. In the newborn, seizures recur frequently up to the seventh day and then infrequently for weeks or months. The outcome is favourable, with only a small number developing mild epilepsy later.

During the early months of life, epileptic seizures are uncommon, partial, fragmented and difficult to recognize. They may be a warning sign of serious neurodevelopmental abnormality. *Early infantile epileptic encephalopathy* or Ohtahara's syndrome presents early and is characterized by tonic spasms, psychomotor retardation and a typical burst–suppression EEG pattern. The prognosis is uniformly bad. The condition may be familial and occurs in association with major brain malformations and metabolic defects, especially non-ketotic hyperglycinaemia (Ohtahara, 1984).

Pyridoxine (vitamin B₆) deficiency, transmitted as an autosomal recessive trait, is a rare disorder caused by defective binding of pyridoxine to its apoenzyme, glutamate decarboxylase. The production of the inhibitory neurotransmitter GABA is impaired as a result. Continuous seizures, usually beginning within hours of birth and unresponsive to antiepileptic drugs, occur and are abolished by pyridoxine given intravenously. The diagnosis should be considered in any young infant with intractable seizures (Bankier et al, 1983) and indeed in every infant up to 18 months who presents with severe generalized or even partial seizures without obvious cause (Goutières and Aicardi, 1985).

Three months to 4 years

During this period of life the seizure threshold is low and reactive seizures, especially with fever, are common. Febrile convulsions are age-related and consist of generalized tonic–clonic seizures, which are usually brief and the result of a viral illness. A small proportion of attacks is prolonged and potentially brain-damaging. Recurrence is likely in one third of cases. Essentially, this is a benign disorder with an absolute risk of developing later epilepsy of 2–4% (O'Donohoe, 1992b).

Several important epileptic syndromes may occur during this epoch but they are relatively uncommon. *West's syndrome of infantile spasms* usually begins between 4 and 7 months, is commoner in boys and is characterized by repetitive flexor or extensor spasms or both, by arrest of psychomotor development and by a grossly disorganized EEG pattern (hypsarrhythmia). The condition described by West (1841) refers to a small group of patients whose previous neurodevelopmental progress has been normal and in whom there is no identifiable aetiology. In these *cryptogenic* cases, numbering only about 15% of the total (Hrachovy and Frost, 1989), there may be a good response to adrenocorticotrophic hormone (ACTH), with cessation of spasms and resumption of normal development. The great majority of cases, however, arising in children with suspected or identifiable structural pathology in the brain, especially tuberous sclerosis, show no such response to ACTH and less than 5% recover (Glaze et al, 1988).

Benign myoclonic epilepsy in infants is a rare epileptic syndrome, characterized by brief bouts of myoclonic jerking, presenting between 6 months and 2 years in otherwise normal children. There is often a family history of epilepsy. Response to treatment and prognosis are good (Dravet et al, 1992). A more sinister syndrome entitled *severe myoclonic epilepsy in infants* presents at 5–6 months of age with severe generalized tonic–clonic or clonic seizures, usually precipitated by fever. Again, there is often a family history of epilepsy and those affected have no previous history of disease or abnormality. Myoclonic seizures follow later, usually after the first birthday. The condition is resistant to treatment and associated with developmental retardation later. No aetiology has been identified but unfavourable genetic factors are thought to be responsible (Aicardi and Gomes, 1989).

The *Lennox–Gastaut syndrome* presents between 1 and 8 years, usually before 5 years of age. A variety of seizures and drop attacks are characteristic. Atypical prolonged absences and episodes of minor epileptic status are usual and there is associated mental retardation. The EEG characteristically shows slow spike-wave complexes and also fast discharges during sleep. In the majority, the syndrome develops in a setting of previous abnormality including, in some cases, previous infantile spasms, and investigations show structural changes in the brain. However, about 30% of cases must be regarded as cryptogenic since they involve previously normal children. Whether symptomatic or cryptogenic, the outcome is very unfavourable with 80–90% showing mental impairment, often with intractable epilepsy (Kurokawa et al, 1980).

Epilepsy in which myoclonic jerks are the most characteristic feature may present in normal children from 6 months to 6 years. There may be associated afebrile or febrile tonic–clonic seizures. Entitled *true or cryptogenic myoclonic epilepsy of children*, the condition has an unpredictable course but the outcome is invariably better than in the Lennox–Gastaut syndrome (Aicardi and Gomes, 1989).

Myoclonic–astatic epilepsy is a rare syndrome characterized by a strong genetic predisposition and by epilepsy starting between 1 and 5 years in previously normal children. The attacks involve an initial myoclonus of the arms followed by an abrupt loss of muscle tone and precipitate falling to the ground. Myoclonic jerks, absences and other seizures also occur but there are no tonic seizures or tonic drop attacks as in the Lennox–Gastaut syndrome. The response to therapy and prognosis are also better than in that condition. There is, however, an overlap with other myoclonic epilepsies, including the Lennox–Gastaut syndrome, and differential diagnosis can be difficult (Doose, 1992).

Four to ten years

In this period, there is a predominance of primary or idiopathic generalized and partial epilepsies. The first of these is *childhood absence epilepsy*, now the preferred term for petit mal. Presenting at 6–7 years, it shows a strong genetic predisposition and girls are more frequently affected. The absences are usually brief with sudden cessation of activity and a blank stare but there may be slight clonic movements and mild automatisms. Hyperventilation may provoke an attack. Characteristic regular spike-wave complexes are present in the EEG. The prognosis is usually favourable with up to 80% achieving permanent remission (Cavazzuti, 1980). It is less good when generalized tonic–clonic seizures also occur and there may then be a recurrence of grand mal epilepsy during adolescence (Loiseau et al, 1983b).

Epilepsy with myoclonic absences is a related but much rarer syndrome. It usually begins at about 7 years and there are frequent daily absences accompanied by severe bilateral rhythmic myoclonus, particularly involving the shoulders, arms and face. It is commoner in males. The EEG is similar to that of childhood absence epilepsy but the condition is much more drug-resistant. Some patients undergo mental deterioration combined with worsening of the epilepsy (Tassinari et al, 1992).

Generalized tonic–clonic seizures (grand mal) are the commonest of all convulsive manifestations in childhood and, as the presenting symptoms of a primary generalized epilepsy, may occur at any age. A common presentation is between 5 and 11 years, when the condition is called *childhood grand mal*. Genetic influences are strong and the affected child is, as a rule, otherwise normal. As with childhood absence epilepsy, the EEG shows regular spike-wave complexes and the response to medication is excellent with remission taking place in over 90% (Todt, 1984). As already mentioned, the co-existence of absence seizures implies a less favourable prognosis, and those patients with onset during adolescence do less well. Generalized tonic–clonic seizures may also occur in this age group and also during adolescence in *photosensitive epilepsy*, a condition in which attacks are usually produced by close television viewing. Attacks are generally infrequent and remission of inherited photosensitivity may be expected early in the third decade (Jeavons et al, 1986).

The Landau–Kleffner syndrome with epilepsy or *acquired aphasia of childhood with epilepsy* is a rare condition beginning between 2 and 8 years. The first symptom may be aphasia or epilepsy. The aphasia is due to auditory verbal agnosia, an inability to comprehend spoken language. Spontaneous speech diminishes or is lost and the patient appears deaf. Seizures, either generalized or partial, occur in two thirds of patients. Reactive behavioural changes are common but intelligence is unimpaired. Epileptic discharges occur predominantly in the temporal areas in the EEG. There may be diagnostic confusion with deafness, autism and juvenile psychosis. The seizures are infrequent and usually remit. The aphasia may resolve after weeks or months, or may partially improve. Some cases show an improvement following ACTH therapy. The older the child at the time of onset the better the prognosis. With onset before the age of 5 years, the outlook for full recovery is poor (Gordon, 1990).

Another rare and probably related syndrome is that of *electrical status epilepticus during slow sleep* (ESES syndrome) which is characterized by partial and generalized motor seizures, mainly during sleep, beginning usually at 4–5 years and diagnosed by the finding of remarkable continuous spike-wave activity in the EEG during deep sleep. Psychomotor development before onset may be normal or abnormal but, in either situation, the condition usually leads to a slow decline in intellectual and language functioning and to disturbances of memory and of temporospatial orientation. Antiepileptic drugs are usually ineffective and the duration of the syndrome is variable. However, there is a prospect of remission during adolescence (Yasuhara et al, 1991).

Partial or localization-related epilepsies are disorders in which seizure symptomatology and investigations indicate a localized origin of the seizures. Primary partial epilepsies are age-related, apparently non-lesional and subject to spontaneous remission. They occur in otherwise normal children of normal intelligence who may have a family history of a similar epilepsy. The seizures are usually brief and infrequent and, although seizure patterns may vary, they are usually constant for an individual patient. The most frequently occurring of these epilepsies is the syndrome of *benign partial epilepsy with centrotemporal spikes*, also known as *rolandic epilepsy*. This very common disorder accounts for 15–20% of children with epilepsy, and is particularly common in the age group 5–15 years. It occurs, in fact, four times as frequently as childhood absence epilepsy. An aphorism that aptly describes this syndrome is that the seizures appear during the first decade and disappear during the second. The usual age of presentation is 6–10 years. The seizure type consists of unilateral paraesthesias and/or tonic or clonic convulsions involving the face, lips, tongue, and pharyngeal and laryngeal muscles. Speech arrest and drooling may occur. Consciousness is preserved as is usual in a simple partial seizure. After the attack, the child describes sensations of numbness and tingling in lips, tongue and cheek on one side and sometimes in the ipsilateral arm also. The attack may evolve into a secondarily generalized tonic–clonic seizure. This rarely happens during waking but is a common outcome during sleep, when the seizure discharges are activated greatly. Nocturnal seizures are commoner in younger patients and hemifacial attacks are more frequent in older children. The EEG shows typical unilateral or bilateral centrotemporal spikes which occur very frequently in sleep recordings. The prognosis is excellent, with or without antiepileptic drug therapy, and universal and permanent remission occurs by the mid-teens at the latest (Holmes, 1992).

There is a much rarer syndrome entitled *benign partial epilepsy with occipital paroxysms*, in which repetitive occipital spiking occurs on eye closure. Seizures commence with visual symptoms, followed by motor or psychomotor manifestations and sometimes by a migraine headache. The condition is more drug resistant than the previous disorder but eventual remission can be expected during adolescence (Panayiotopoulos, 1989).

Secondary or symptomatic partial epilepsies are of great importance at all times of life and are characterized by simple or complex partial seizures. Complex partial seizures, secondary to structural changes in the temporal or frontal areas and involving the limbic system, may commence at any time in infancy or childhood but become more clearly defined in the epoch of 4–10 years. They account for up to 25% of all childhood seizures and are often difficult to recognize and treat; however, they are increasingly amenable to surgical treatment (Wyllie and Lüders, 1989; Enlow and Moshé, 1991; Wyllie, 1991).

An important though rare epileptic syndrome that presents with simple partial seizures or, more often, with partial epileptic status continuing for prolonged periods and usually involving a distal limb is *epilepsia partialis continua*. Two types are recognized, one beginning before 2 years and associated with a non-progressive lesion of central location and a second, with a median age of onset of 5 years, in which the partial motor seizures become progressively worse and there is also progressive neurological and intellectual deterioration. The second variety, also known as *Rasmussen's syndrome*, is thought to be due to a chronic localized viral encephalitis, although no organisms have been identified (Rasmussen and Andermann, 1989).

From 9–10 years onwards

The primary generalized and partial epilepsies described in the preceding section may present for the first time at this period of late childhood and adolescence, and epilepsy related to temporal lobe pathology and character-ized by complex partial seizures becomes an even more important and serious problem. Although slow-growing *cerebral tumours* are a relatively rare cause of partial epilepsies during childhood and adolescence, they should always be considered as a diagnostic possibility in resistant seizure disorders at any age (Lee et al, 1989).

A syndrome of *benign partial epilepsy during adolescence* has been described, mainly in otherwise normal boys. The onset is usually at 13–14 years and the attacks may be simple or complex partial seizures, often with secondary generalization. A single unexplained seizure may be the only clinical event in 80% of cases, or there may be a cluster of attacks over 24–36 h. The EEG is usually normal or shows non-specific abnormalities, and the prognosis is excellent. A cerebral tumour is often suspected as a cause but the diagnosis is easily eliminated by brain scanning (Loiseau et al, 1983a).

An important epileptic syndrome during this epoch is that entitled *juvenile myoclonic epilepsy* or the *Janz syndrome*. It is now considered to constitute 7–9% of all life-time epilepsies and to be the commonest primary epilepsy presenting during adolescence. The cardinal symptom is the occurrence at or soon after awakening of brief bilateral synchronous jerks of shoulders and arms, often occurring in clusters and unassociated with loss of consciousness (unlike epilepsy with myoclonic absences). The patient may throw down objects that he or she is holding (the 'flying cornflakes' syndrome). A minority of patients may fall suddenly. Triggering factors for attacks include lack of sleep, sudden and unexpected arousal from sleep and excessive alcohol consumption. The majority of those affected go on to develop generalized tonic–clonic seizures, also on awakening, after an interval of 1–3 years, and a small number also have absences. Some demonstrate photosensitivity. Intelligence is unimpaired and investigations are generally negative apart from the EEG which shows polyspike and wave discharges against a normal background activity (Janz, 1989). Genetic linkage studies have indicated a probable association with an abnormality in chromosome 6, at least in certain family studies (Delgado-Escueta et al, 1989). The prognosis of this syndrome is very favourable if it is treated early and consistently and if the patient is prepared to make modifications to his or her way of life. However, although the response to suitable medication is usually encouraging, the likelihood of being cured with drugs is slight since relapses occur in 75–100% of patients following reduction in drug dosage or discontinuation of therapy, even after years of freedom from seizures. In the majority of patients, therefore, treatment must be life-long.

Epilepsy with grand mal on awakening may occur as an isolated epileptic syndrome during adolescence, often associated with photosensitivity. Triggering factors for seizures are the same as those for the Janz syndrome, and girls may report an increased seizure frequency just before or during menstruation. There may be a second peak of seizure occurrence in the evening. The prognosis is good with treatment but, as in the previous disorder, relapse occurs if treatment is omitted or stopped (Wolf, 1992).

SUMMARY

The modern era of seizure classification dates from 1969. Seizures were classified into partial and generalized. The classification was revised in 1981 when a more flexible categorization was adopted, especially of partial seizures, to allow for the dynamic evolution of individual seizures from one type into another and also to take account of the disturbances of consciousness and memory that are associated with complex partial seizures.

Classifications of the epilepsies have also been developed and during the 1980s an International Classification was devised dividing them into generalized epilepsies, presenting mainly with generalized seizures, and partial or localization-related epilepsies, presenting predominantly with partial seizures, implying a definable localization in the cortex. A further division was made into those epilepsies with known aetiology (symptomatic or secondary) and those with no known aetiology (idiopathic or primary).

During the past two decades it has also been possible to identify many individual epileptic syndromes occurring during infancy, childhood and adolescence, of which individual seizures are but one manifestation. The syndromic approach has led to more precise diagnostic, therapeutic and prognostic attitudes to the patient with epilepsy, has improved communication and exchange of ideas about epilepsy and has led to more rational use of antiepileptic drugs.

Nevertheless, the concept of epileptic syndromes does not embrace all forms of convulsive disorder and other methods of categorization are also employed in conjunction with the syndromic method. These include the neurobiological approach in which attempts are made to build a profile of the patient based on clinical, EEG and neuropsychological data.

A chronological framework for the clinical subdivision of the childhood epilepsies and epileptic syndromes is one that has particular appeal for the paediatrician. Four epochs, ranging from infancy through early and late childhood and continuing into adolescence, are recognized. This method has been used in this chapter to provide brief descriptions of the important epileptic syndromes occurring in the paediatric population.

REFERENCES

Aicardi J (1986) *Epilepsy in Children*, pp 6–7. New York: Raven Press.
Aicardi J (1992) Epilepsy and inborn errors of metabolism. In Roger J, Bureau M, Dravet C et al (eds) *Epileptic Syndromes in Infancy, Childhood and Adolescence*, 2nd edn, pp 97–102. London: John Libbey.
Aicardi J & Gomes AL (1989) The myoclonic epilepsies of childhood. *Cleveland Clinic Journal of Medicine* **56 (supplement):** 34–39.
American Academy of Neurology (1989) Assessment: intensive EEG video monitoring for epilepsy. *Neurology* **39:** 1101–1102.
Bankier A, Turner M & Hopkins IJ (1983) Pyridoxine dependent seizures: a wider clinical spectrum. *Archives of Disease in Childhood* **58:** 415–418.
Berkovic SF, Andermann F, Andermann E & Gloor P (1987) Concepts of absence epilepsies. Discrete syndromes or biological continuum? *Neurology* **37:** 993–1000.
Cavazzuti GB (1980) Epidemiology of different types of epilepsy in school age children in Modena, Italy. *Epilepsia* **21:** 57–62.
Commission on Classification and Terminology of the International League Against Epilepsy (1981) Proposal for revised clinical and electroencephalographic classification of epileptic seizures. *Epilepsia* **22:** 489–501.
Commission on Classification and Terminology of the International League Against Epilepsy (1989) Proposal for classification of epilepsies and epileptic syndromes. *Epilepsia* **30:** 389–399.
Delgado-Escueta AV, Greenberg DA, Treiman L et al (1989) Mapping the gene for juvenile myoclonic epilepsy. *Epilepsia* **30 (supplement 4):** S8–S18.
Doose H (1992) Myoclonic–astatic epilepsy. In Degen RE & Dreifuss FE (eds) *Benign Localized and Generalized Epilepsies of Early Childhood. Epilepsy Research Supplement*, no. 6, pp 163–168. Amsterdam: Elsevier.
Dravet C, Bureau M & Roger J (1992) Benign myoclonic epilepsy in infants. In Roger J, Bureau M, Dravet C et al (eds) *Epileptic Syndromes in Infancy, Childhood and Adolescence*, 2nd edn, pp 67–74. London: John Libbey.
Dreifuss FE (1990) The epilepsies: clinical implications of the International Classification. *Epilepsia* **31 (supplement 3):** S3–S10.
Enlow TC & Moshé SL (1991) Pediatric epilepsy. *Current Opinion in Pediatrics* **3:** 944–949.
Gastaut H (1970) Clinical and electroencephalographical classification of epileptic seizures. *Epilepsia* **10 (supplement):** 2–21.
Glaze DJ, Hrachovy RA, Frost JD et al (1988) Prospective study of outcome of infants with infantile spasms treated during controlled studies of ACTH and prednisone. *Journal of Pediatrics* **12:** 389–396.
Gordon N (1990) Acquired aphasia in childhood: the Landau–Kleffner syndrome. *Developmental Medicine and Child Neurology* **32:** 267–274.
Goutières F & Aicardi J (1985) Atypical presentations of pyridoxine-dependent seizures: a treatable cause of intractable epilepsy in infants. *Annals of Neurology* **17:** 117–120.

Holmes GL (1989) Electroencephalographic and neuroradiologic evaluation of children with epilepsy. *Pediatric Clinics of North America* **32(2):** 395–420.

Holmes GL (1992) Rolandic epilepsy: clinical and electroencephalographic features. In Degen R & Dreifuss FE (eds) *Benign Localized and Generalized Epilepsies of Early Childhood. Epilepsy Research Supplement*, no. 6, pp 29–44. Amsterdam: Elsevier.

Hrachovy RA & Frost JD (1989) Infantile spasms. *Cleveland Clinical Journal of Medicine* **56 (supplement):** S.10–S.16.

Janz D (1989) Juvenile myoclonic epilepsy: epilepsy with impulsive petit mal. *Cleveland Clinic Journal of Medicine* **56 (supplement):** S23–S33.

Jeavons PM, Bishop A & Harding GFA (1986) The prognosis of photosensitivity. *Epilepsia* **27:** 569–575.

Kurokawa T, Goya N, Fukayama Y et al (1980) West syndrome and Lennox–Gastaut syndrome: a survey of natural history. *Pediatrics* **61:** 81–88.

Lee TKY, Nakasu Y, Jeffree MA et al (1989) Indolent glioma: a cause of epilepsy. *Archives of Disease in Childhood* **64:** 1666–1671.

Leppert M, Anderson VE, Quattlebaum T et al (1989) Benign familial neonatal convulsions linked to genetic markers on chromosome 20. *Nature* **337:** 647–648.

Loiseau P, Dartigues JF & Pestre M (1983a) Prognosis of partial epileptic seizures in the adolescent. *Epilepsia* **24:** 472–481.

Loiseau P, Pestre M, Dartigues JF et al (1983b) Long-term prognosis in two forms of childhood epilepsy: typical absence seizures and epilepsy with rolandic (centrotemporal) EEG foci. *Annals of Neurology* **13:** 642–648.

Manford M, Hart YM, Sander JWAS & Shorvon SD (1992) The national general practice study of epilepsy: the syndromic classification of the International League Against Epilepsy applied to epilepsy in a general population. *Archives of Neurology* **49:** 801–808.

Moshé SL (1987) Epileptogenesis and the immature brain. *Epilepsia* **28 (supplement 1):** S3–S15.

O'Donohoe NV (1991) The epilepsies. In Eyre J & Boyd R (eds) *Paediatric Specialty Practice for the 1990s*, pp 51–64. London: Royal College of Physicians of London.

O'Donohoe NV (1992a) Delineation of epileptic syndromes. *Current Paediatrics* **2:** 68–72.

O'Donohoe NV (1992b) Febrile convulsions. In Roger J, Bureau M, Dravet C et al (eds) *Epileptic Syndromes in Infancy, Childhood and Adolescence*, 2nd edn, pp 45–52. London: John Libbey.

Ohtahara S (1984) Seizure disorders in infancy and childhood. *Brain and Development* **6:** 509–519.

Panayiotopoulos CP (1989) Benign childhood epilepsy with occipital paroxysms. A 15 year prospective study. *Annals of Neurology* **26:** 51–56.

Pryor DS, Don N & Macourt DC (1981) Fifth-day fits: a syndrome of neonatal convulsions. *Archives of Disease in Childhood* **56:** 753–758.

Rasmussen T & Andermann F (1989) Update on the syndrome of 'chronic encephalitis' and epilepsy. *Cleveland Clinic Journal of Medicine* **56 (supplement):** S181–S184.

Roger J, Bureau M, Dravet C et al (eds) (1992) *Epileptic Syndromes in Infancy, Childhood and Adolescence*, 2nd edn. London: John Libbey.

Scher MS & Painter MJ (1989) Controversies concerning neonatal seizures. *Pediatric Clinics of North America* **36:** 281–310.

Tassinari CA, Bureau M & Thomas P (1992) Epilepsy with myoclonic absences. In Roger J, Bureau M, Dravet C et al (eds) *Epileptic Syndromes in Infancy, Childhood and Adolescence*, 2nd edn, pp 151–160. London: John Libbey.

Taylor J, Holmes G & Walshe FMR (eds) (1931) *Selected Writings of John Hughlings Jackson*, vol. 1, p 8. London: Hodder & Stoughton.

Todt H (1984) The late prognosis of epilepsy in childhood: results of a prospective follow-up study. *Epilepsia* **25:** 137–144.

West WJ (1841) On a peculiar form of infantile convulsions. *Lancet* **i:** 724–725.

Wolf P (1992) Epilepsy with grand mal on awakening. In Roger J, Bureau M, Dravet C et al (eds) *Epileptic Syndromes in Infancy, Childhood and Adolescence*, 2nd edn, pp 329–342. London: John Libbey.

Wyllie E (1991) Cortical resection for children with epilepsy. *American Journal of Diseases of Children* **145:** 314–320.

484

Wyllie E & Lüders H (1989) Complex partial seizures in children: clinical manifestations and identification of surgical candidates. *Cleveland Clinical Journal of Medicine* **56 (supplement):** S43–S52.

Yasuhara A, Yoshida H, Hatanaka T et al (1991) Epilepsy with continuous spike-waves during slow sleep and its treatment. *Epilepsia* **32:** 59–62.

3

Principles of genetic counselling in the childhood epilepsies

SHIRLEY V. HODGSON
CHRISTOPHER M. VERITY

Although it is 2500 years since Hippocrates suggested that epilepsy was inherited, until recently geneticists thought that epilepsy was too complex to deal with. Why is the subject so difficult? The source of the difficulty can be summed up in one word—heterogeneity. Not only are the epilepsies a clinically heterogeneous group of disorders but within individual types of epilepsy there is also genetic heterogeneity.

Clinical heterogeneity

Epilepsy is not a disease, it is the state of having recurrent afebrile seizures. This state can have many different causes. Most seizures do not consist of a single sign or symptom: they are a stereotyped symptom complex (Wolf, 1991). Often seizures occur in characteristic clinical settings as part of recognizable epileptic syndromes. Attempts have been made to classify seizure types and epileptic syndromes on a rational basis (Commission on Classification and Terminology of the International League Against Epilepsy, 1989; see Chapter 2). This has brought ordered thinking to a complex subject and facilitated the study of the genetics of the epilepsies.

Genetic heterogeneity

A similar clinical phenotype can result from mutations at different genetic loci. Also, different mutations within a single locus can be associated with variable clinical manifestations. Environmental factors may be entirely responsible for particular cases or they may modify the phenotype. It is therefore not surprising that there is evidence for genetic heterogeneity in the epilepsies (Anderson et al, 1991b). Seizures can occur as a result of a number of structural or functional abnormalities, each of which may be subject to genetic influence.

How important is the study of the genetics of epilepsy to the practising clinician? The well-defined clinical syndromes causing epilepsy account for only a small proportion of cases and the single-gene defects that are associated with seizures account for less than 1% of all the epilepsies

Baillière's Clinical Paediatrics—
Vol. 2, No. 3, August 1994
ISBN 0–7020–1862–7

(Shorvon, 1991). Therefore, in the majority of children with epilepsy, there is no clear genetic cause. However, this is an area of rapid change and of increasing practical importance, as a number of excellent reviews have recently shown (Gardiner, 1990; Anderson et al, 1991a; Whitehouse and Gardiner, 1991; Noebels, 1992). We therefore start this chapter with a summary of the evidence that heredity is an important factor in the genesis of the epilepsies. We then discuss the principles of genetics as applied to the epilepsies of childhood. This is followed by a practical guide to the assessment of genetic risk. We conclude by attempting to look into the future of a rapidly changing subject.

EVIDENCE THAT MANY OF THE EPILEPSIES ARE INHERITED

Evidence resulting from the classification of seizures and epileptic syndromes

A major division of the epilepsies is into those that are symptomatic of an immediate or remote cause and those that are idiopathic, i.e. they are isolated phenomena without a known underlying cause other than a possible hereditary predisposition. Some of the symptomatic epilepsies are known to have a genetic cause: about 160 monogenic (single-gene) defects are associated with seizures (Anderson et al, 1991b).

Epidemiological studies report less familial aggregation in partial than in generalized epilepsy; however, relatives of patients with partial seizures appear to have a higher seizure risk than relatives of controls, suggesting that genetic factors are important in at least some partial epilepsies (Ottman, 1989).

Much work has gone into the classification of seizure types. In addition, it is increasingly recognized that there are specific epileptic syndromes (Commission on Classification and Terminology of the International League Against Epilepsy, 1989). Some of these epileptic syndromes may have an underlying genetic basis, as is discussed below.

Epidemiological evidence

In epidemiology, the unit of study is the population, not the patient. It is important to determine the expected frequency of epilepsy in the general population. The most important measure of this for genetic studies is the cumulative incidence (DeLorenzo, 1991). This is the summation of the age-specific incidences to determine the proportion of the population that has been affected by a certain age. The cumulative incidence is particularly important in the study of the epilepsies of childhood because many of them are strikingly age-dependent. Unfortunately point-prevalence rates are more easily obtained than incidence rates (Shorvon, 1991). Most studies quote a point prevalence of epilepsy of 4–10 per 1000 population. There seem to be no major differences between different populations so it is difficult to define aetiological influences by comparing them. Case–control methods have rarely been used in epidemiological studies; it is possible that they would reveal hitherto unsuspected aetiologies (Shorvon, 1991).

Population-based studies have served to correct distorted views of aetiology that result from the study of selected groups of patients attending specialized hospitals or clinics. For instance, histories obtained from adults undergoing temporal lobectomy for intractable seizures suggested that febrile convulsions were an important cause of mesial temporal sclerosis, which thus led to intractable epilepsy (Falconer et al, 1964). A population-based study of a cohort of children provided evidence that if this sequence of events occurs it does so rarely (Verity and Golding, 1991).

Family studies

These have been the basis for the investigation of the genetics of epilepsy (Anderson et al, 1991b). Early family studies were of epilepsies in general and of relatives in general. Then, defined seizure types and associated EEG patterns were studied in specific groups of relatives, as shown below. The results of family studies depend in part on whether or not EEG findings in asymptomatic family members are included in the analysis (Gardiner, 1990).

Twin studies are a useful form of family study. Anderson and co-workers (1989) combined the results of six major twin studies and found that the concordance rate for epilepsy was 60% for monozygotic twins compared with 13% for dizygotic twins. These studies provide good evidence that genetic factors have a role in the development of some seizures. Twins have been used to study febrile convulsions (Tsuboi and Endo, 1991) and specific types of epilepsy (Anderson et al, 1991b).

The findings of some family studies of individual seizure types are summarized below.

Generalized-onset epilepsy

The approach is exemplified in the papers of Metrakos and Metrakos, which are classics in the field. They investigated probands with either grand mal or absence epilepsy and generalized spike and wave on the EEG and found that the risk of seizures among siblings of probands was 12.7% compared with 4.7% among siblings of controls (Metrakos and Metrakos, 1960, 1961). They also studied EEG abnormalities in siblings and suggested that there was an autosomal dominant inheritance for the underlying EEG abnormality (Metrakos and Metrakos, 1974). More recently Anderman (1982) concluded that the hypothesis of polygenic inheritance fitted the data better.

Doose et al (1973) studied 239 children with absence epilepsy. They recorded the EEGs of siblings and control children. In 30% of families at least one relative had a history of seizures. The highest incidence of seizures was in siblings (7%) and parents (6%). The incidence was higher in the families of female than of male probands. The EEGs of the siblings showed θ rhythms, spike-wave patterns or photosensitivity in 28%. Spike waves at rest and during hyperventilation were found in up to 20% of siblings, depending on age: the maximum incidence in controls was 3%. These results were thought to favour polygenic inheritance of epilepsies with spike-wave absences rather than autosomal dominant inheritance.

Doose and Baier (1987a) studied genetic factors in epilepsies with primary generalized minor seizures (absences, myoclonic and myoclonic–astatic seizures, partly in combination with generalized tonic–clonic attacks). The study included 400 children and 4514 relatives. When the whole sample was studied the incidence of seizures of any type among siblings and parents was 6%. Siblings of male and female probands were almost equally affected. Mothers' siblings reported seizures more often than fathers' siblings.

Janz and Christian described 'impulsive petit mal' in 1957. This was later known as juvenile myoclonic epilepsy. It is a syndrome of idiopathic generalized epilepsy which starts around puberty and includes myoclonic jerks, generalized tonic–clonic seizures and absences. Tsuboi and Christian (1973) studied 319 probands with 'impulsive petit mal' and 1618 first-degree relatives. Of these relatives, 66 (4%) were epileptic; their seizure types included generalized tonic–clonic, impulsive petit mal and absences. In general, the incidence of epilepsy was higher among relatives of female probands than among those of male probands, and the risk of epilepsy was higher among female than male relatives.

Ottman and colleagues (1985) reviewed the literature and found agreement that the offspring of epileptic women had a higher risk of epilepsy than those of epileptic men. The possible mechanisms are discussed below in the section dealing with mitochondrial inheritance.

Partial epilepsies

Between 37% and 66% of the childhood epilepsies are partial epilepsies, depending on the age range and the method of recruitment of cases (Dalla Bernardina et al, 1992). Authors studying the different forms of idiopathic partial epilepsy of childhood report a high proportion with a family history of epilepsy. Bray and Wiser (1965) studied 40 probands with partial epilepsy whose EEGs showed paroxysmal sharp waves or spikes in the mid-temporal region and suggested that there was autosomal dominant inheritance of the trait with age-related penetrance. Similar conclusions were reached by Heijbel et al (1975) who studied 19 probands with 'benign epilepsy of childhood and centrotemporal EEG foci (rolandic discharges)'—the syndrome had by then been more formally delineated. They found that of 34 siblings 15% had seizures and rolandic discharges and 19% had rolandic discharges alone. Of 38 parents, 11% had a history of seizures in childhood but not adulthood and only one parent had rolandic discharges on the EEG.

Recently Doose and Baier (1991) pointed out that there is a group of childhood epilepsies that have two common characteristics: a focal or multifocal origin and a favourable prognosis. This group includes benign partial epilepsy with centrotemporal sharp waves, atypical benign partial epilepsy, benign partial epilepsy with affective symptoms and benign partial epilepsy with occipital paroxysms. They performed a study of 57 sibships with focal sharp waves of genetic origin and found that pairs of relatives who shared the EEG characteristics of focal and multifocal sharp waves showed a broad spectrum of epileptic and non-epileptic conditions, ranging from mild selective performance deficits to complex psychometric retardation, from simple rolandic epilepsy to severe epilepsies with minor seizures or bio-electric status. Thus there appears to be an underlying 'focal liability' which may be associated with a wide range of phenotypes. They suggest that the marked age dependence of the symptoms and the disappearance of both seizures and EEG abnormalities at puberty justify the use of the term 'hereditary impairment of brain maturation', possibly transmitted by an autosomal dominant gene.

Febrile convulsions

According to Tsuboi and Endo (1991) a number of different modes of inheritance have been suggested for this relatively common problem of childhood: simple autosomal dominant, autosomal recessive or multi-factorial. In 1991 they presented an analysis of twin and family data that provides some support for a multifactorial model of inheritance.

Major conclusions that have come from family studies

Anderson and co-workers (1991b) have summarized the 'state of the art':

1. The sibling and offspring risks for seizures are usually higher when the proband has a younger age at onset.
2. The seizure phenotype in affected siblings and offspring is skewed toward that in probands, but the correspondence is not exact.
3. Interictal EEG abnormalities may be part of the phenotype and may be closer to gene action than seizures, but the specific EEG patterns are not predictable.
4. There is good evidence for genetic heterogeneity.
5. Seizure risks are higher for the offspring and siblings of female than of male probands.
6. Gene mapping is possible.
7. Empirical risk data are available for genetic counselling.

Animal studies

'The search for human epilepsy genes can be greatly facilitated by parallel studies of epileptic phenotypes in other species' (Noebels, 1991). Neuro-logical mutant mice have been extensively used as a large number of inbred strains and mapped neurological mutants are available.

The inherited convulsive disorders in mice were reviewed by Seyfried and Glaser (1985) and Seyfried et al (1986). The disorders include audiogenic seizures, the epilepsy (E1) mouse, various spontaneous seizures, the tottering–leaner syndrome, seizures associated with cerebellar abnor-malities, seizures associated with myelin disorders and alcohol withdrawal seizures. For many major types of epilepsy in humans there is a counterpart in mice. The authors used mice that were susceptible to audiogenic seizures. They studied inbred and congenic mouse strains and were able to identify a major gene, *Ias*, that inhibits the spread of seizure activity. They also found that juvenile-onset and adult-onset audiogenic seizures in the mouse are controlled by different genetic systems (Seyfried et al, 1986). The juvenile-onset seizure susceptibility was found to be associated with Ca^{2+} ATPase deficiency in recombinant inbred mice. A deficiency of Ca^{2+} ATPase activity could cause defective synaptic transmission. This was the first description of the inheritance of a neurochemical trait together with an idiopathic convulsive disorder and it could be an important basic mechanism of epilepsy.

More recently Qiauo and Noebels (1991) studied two mouse mutants—the tottering and stargazer mutants—and revealed the existence of two distinct and independent neurochemical mechanisms in the two mutants that produce the same 'endpoint', inherited spike-wave epilepsy. The homozygous tottering mutants show hyperplasia of central noradrenergic axons originating in the locus coeruleus. In contrast the stargazer mutants show no alterations in noradrenergic fibre innervation.

Several mouse mutants have been mapped to different chromosomes and other 'modifier' genes have been mapped that influence the epilepsy phenotype (Rise et al, 1991). These examples show how animal studies have provided evidence for the existence of epilepsy genes and have given important insights into possible underlying mechanisms of seizure disorders.

PRINCIPLES OF GENETIC COUNSELLING IN THE EPILEPSIES

Monogenic (single-gene) defects

A large number of monogenic defects are known to be associated with seizures (Bird, 1987; Blandfort et al, 1987). The mechanisms causing seizures in each syndrome probably differ.

Autosomal dominant disorders

The best-known examples are neurofibromatosis and tuberous sclerosis, both neurocutaneous disorders with a variable phenotype, where focal abnormalities in the brain may trigger seizures. These conditions are manifest clinically when the abnormal gene is present on only one of a pair of alleles, the other being normal (i.e. the individual is heterozygous for the abnormal gene) and an affected individual has a 50:50 risk of passing the disorder to each child. The risk to apparently normal parents of having a second child with the disorder should be low, as the disorder probably arose as the result of a new mutation in the affected child. However, careful examination may reveal minimal clinical features of the disorder in one of the parents, indicating that they are affected and at 50% risk of handing their condition on to their offspring. This has been documented recently for tuberous sclerosis in family studies (Osborne, 1988). In addition there is a possibility that one parent may have a mosaic cell line in their germ cells, with or without involvement of somatic cells, so that they could show features of the disease in only a part of their body (Riccardi and Eichner, 1986); these individuals may be at risk of having further affected offspring.

Juvenile-onset Huntington's disease is associated with seizures in about 50% of cases (Hayden, 1981). Interestingly, the early-onset form of this disease usually occurs when the condition is inherited from the father, a possible example of genetic imprinting (Reik, 1988); see below. The Ramsay Hunt syndrome, with myoclonus and ataxia, is genetically heterogeneous, but in some families appears to be inherited as an autosomal dominant (Harding, 1989).

Autosomal recessive disorders

There are many autosomal recessive disorders associated with epilepsy. These are manifested only in individuals who are homozygous for the mutant gene, i.e. both their alleles are mutant, usually meaning that they have inherited the faulty gene from both parents, who are therefore carriers. The parents are usually phenotypically normal and have a one in four chance of having another affected child with the same partner. Consanguineous marriages are more likely to result in offspring with recessive disorders since the parents are more likely to share common genes than non-consanguineous parents.

In some autosomal recessive conditions the predisposition to seizures may be due to the accumulation of toxic metabolites resulting from a metabolic block, as in phenylketonuria, and appropriate treatment of the metabolic imbalance may reduce or abolish the seizures. In other cases there may be a defect in neurotransmitter metabolism, as in pyridoxine-dependent seizures. Abnormal transport or absorption of factors required for CNS functioning may be responsible for seizures in abetalipoproteinaemia. Storage diseases (particularly the lipid storage diseases) may be associated with neurological regression and seizures, and may display characteristic tapetoretinal degeneration (e.g. neuronal ceroid lipofuscinosis) (Francois, 1982). Abnormal cell membrane receptors may cause seizures in genetic forms of myasthenia gravis (Bird, 1987). Myoclonus epilepsy of Unverricht and Lundborg, and a rare condition of epilepsy, dementia and amelogenesis imperfecta, appear also to be inherited as autosomal recessive traits (Christodoulou et al, 1988).

The age of onset of seizures may have diagnostic significance. In non-ketotic hyperglycinaemia and pyridoxine dependency, they may start in the neonate. In phenylketonuria, Tay–Sachs disease and early infantile ceroid lipofuscinosis they start in infancy; in late infantile ceroid lipofuscinosis they start in childhood; in juvenile Gaucher's disease, Spielmeyer–Vogt disease and Lafora disease they start in adolescence; and in Kufs' disease they start in adult life.

X-linked recessive disorders

Characteristically, males manifest these disorders and female carriers do not (or have minimal features). This is because the responsible gene is on the X chromosome. In females there is likely to be a normal allele on their other X chromosome that compensates for the effects of the mutant gene. Males manifest the disease because they only have one X chromosome, which carries the mutant gene in an affected male. If they procreate, all their daughters are carriers and all their sons are unaffected. Female carriers have a 50:50 risk of having affected sons and a 50:50 risk that their daughters will be carriers. Examples of X-linked conditions that are associated with seizures are adrenoleukodystrophy, Menke's syndrome, Lesch–Nyhan disease (hypoxanthine–guanine phosphoribosyltransferase glutamate decarboxylase (HGPRT) deficiency), Lowe's oculocerebrorenal syndrome, a rare X-linked myoclonus epilepsy (Wienker et al, 1979) and the fragile X mental retardation syndrome.

X-linked dominant disorders

Aicardi syndrome, a cause of infantile spasms, is an X-linked dominant disorder expressed in females and probably lethal in the hemizygous male.

Further studies of the mechanisms of seizure development in these disorders should help our understanding of the pathogenesis of epilepsy. Where the metabolic defect is known, and if the responsible enzyme can be assayed in amniotic fluid or chorionic villus cells, prenatal diagnosis may be possible. Linkage analysis or the direct detection of the gene defect (see below) may be used for prenatal testing in conditions where sufficient information is known about the molecular defect underlying the disorder, for example in phenylketonuria.

Chromosomal disorders

Down's syndrome is associated with a risk of epilepsy that increases with age from about 2% below the age of 20 years to 12% after middle age (Veal, 1974; Tangye, 1979). Seizures are described in individuals with trisomy or partial trisomy of chromosomes 13, 18 or 22, and also in Wolf's syndrome (4p−), ring chromosome 14 and partial trisomy 15 (de Grouchy and Turleau, 1984). Trisomy 12p is particularly associated with generalized 3-Hz spike and wave discharges (Guerrini et al, 1990).

Multifactorial inheritance

In this type of inheritance there is an increased incidence of the disorder in the relatives of an index case, but the risk is not as high as would be expected in a monogenic disorder. Neural tube defects provide an example. Other characteristics of this type of inheritance are that the risk is greater to relatives of a severely affected proband, or to relatives of an index case in the less often affected sex (as in Hirschsprung's disease). These phenomena probably indicate an increased genetic predisposition in that family. The supposition is that factors other than the predisposing genes influence the phenotypic expression of these disorders, and one would expect incomplete concordance in affected identical twins, as is observed in epilepsy. Polygenic inheritance means that the phenotypic expression of a disorder is affected by several different genes, each having small additive effects. In the threshold model of multifactorial inheritance it is assumed that the curve of liability has a normal distribution in both the general population and in relatives of an index case, but the curve for relatives is shifted to the right. There is postulated to be a threshold beyond which all individuals are affected. In some conditions there is a sex influence on the susceptibility to develop the phenotype (Carter, 1969; Clarke-Fraser, 1980; Emery and Mueller, 1992).

Mitochondrial inheritance

There is increasing evidence that mutations in the mitochondrial genome cause disease. The inheritance is characteristically maternal: all the offspring of affected females have the disorder (to varying degrees) whereas males do not generally transmit it. This is because the ovum contains some mitochondria, which may be of heterogeneous genotype, but the sperm does not. There are exceptions to this rule; for instance, there are rare conditions showing an autosomal dominant predisposition to mitochondrial genome instability.

The mutations underlying some of these disorders are now being delineated. An A to G transition mutation has been identified as that responsible for the syndrome of myoclonic epilepsy and ragged red fibres (Shoffner et al, 1990). A point mutation in the mitochondrial genome has been found in several unrelated patients with mitochondrial myopathy, encephalopathy, lactic acidosis and stroke-like episodes (MELAS) and not in control subjects (Holt et al, 1989; Wallace, 1989; Kobyashi et al, 1991). There is an increased incidence of seizures in some other mitochondrial encephalomyopathies such as the Kearns–Sayre syndrome (3%), Leigh's disease (31%) and complex I and III deficiencies (DiMauro et al, 1991).

Epidemiological studies consistently report that the offspring of women with epilepsy are more likely to have seizures than those of affected men (Ottman et al, 1988). The multifactorial model of inheritance provides a possible explanation for this observation if it is assumed that males are more susceptible to seizures than females, so that an epileptic female has more of a genetic component to the aetiology of her epilepsy than a male and is therefore more likely to have affected children. However, using this model, more males would be expected to have epilepsy than females overall, which is not what is observed (Leviton and Cowan, 1982; Anderson and Hauser, 1990). A subset of epileptic disorders with mitochondrial inheritance, or a maternal influence on the expression of epilepsy dependent upon the mitochondrial genome, could explain this epidemiological phenomenon. There may be other explanations: mothers may have better recall of seizures in their children than fathers, or a differential in the number of offspring born to epileptic women and men could influence the statistics. Finally, anticonvulsant drugs given to the mother could have an epileptogenic effect on the offspring.

Genomic imprinting

It has become apparent that in some conditions there is a difference in the expression of a genetic disorder depending upon which parent transmitted it. For instance, Huntington's disease is usually more severe when inherited from the father, and autosomal dominantly inherited chemodectomas appear to develop only when the susceptibility gene is inherited from the affected father. Mouse embryos formed entirely from two paternal contributions have been found to develop very poorly although placental development was reasonable, whereas embryos derived from two female components showed relatively good development but had very poor membranes and placentas. A similar phenomenon is seen in humans: hydatidiform moles (with trophoblast hyperplasia and absent fetus) are derived from two paternally derived sets of haploid chromosomes, whereas teratomas, disorganized embryonic tumours with no placental tissue, are derived from two female haploid chromosome contributions. The conclusion from these observations is that there are certain regions of the genome that are expressed differently depending upon the parent that transmitted them, a process known as 'imprinting' (Hall, 1990; Hodgson, 1991; Hodgson and Maher, 1993).

A striking example of the influence of the parental origin of genetic disorders is that of the Prader–Willi and Angelman syndromes. In some cases of both disorders a cytogenetic deletion may be demonstrated in the long arm of chromosome 15 (15q11–q13). This deletion appears similar (although not identical) in both conditions and, if inherited, it is maternally derived in the Angelman syndrome but paternally derived in the Prader–Willi syndrome (Wagstaff et al, 1992). Pedigrees have been reported in which a familial translocation has resulted in the deletion being found in a child with the Prader–Willi syndrome when the defect was inherited from the father and in a child with the Angelman syndrome (in the same extended family) when the defect was inherited from the mother. It has also been shown that the Prader–Willi syndrome may result when there is maternal uniparental disomy, i.e. the child has two copies of the maternal chromosome 15, whereas the Angelman syndrome results from paternal uniparental disomy 15. The presumption is that there is differential expression of maternally and paternally derived genes in this region of chromosome 15. Recent work has identified one such gene, expressed largely in brain and central neurones, which maps to this chromosome region, and in the murine homologue imprinting is assumed to occur as only the male-derived transcript is detected (Hall, 1990; Davies, 1992).

This is of particular interest in the context of epilepsy, since on the whole patients with the Prader–Willi syndrome do not have seizures, while those with the Angelman syndrome do. The specific genes involved in the two conditions are likely to be different, however, and may both be included in deletions large enough to cause either syndrome. One large family has recently been described in which the Angelman syndrome (but not Prader–Willi syndrome) was inherited as an autosomal dominant trait, the condition being expressed only when inherited from the maternal side (Meijers-Heijboer et al, 1992).

APPLICATION OF MOLECULAR GENETIC ANALYSIS TO THE STUDY OF THE EPILEPSIES

DNA can be extracted from any tissue containing nucleated cells and once extracted can be stored so that genetic studies of whole families are possible. Bacterial restriction enzymes recognize specific DNA sequences and can be used to cleave double-stranded DNA at these sites. The resulting series of DNA fragments are of constant size in a given subject but there are variations between individuals because of differences in the DNA sequences. These variations are called restriction fragment length polymorphisms (RFLPs) and can be used as markers for genetic disorders if they are near to or in the gene under investigation. These markers are the basis of the technique of linkage analysis that has been used to search for the genes involved in the causation of various types of epilepsy. Two broad approaches are used. In the first there is a search for linkage between the disease and a few of a library of random polymorphic markers located all over the genome. In the second there is an attempt to establish linkage to 'candidate' genes.

With any linkage strategy there are problems with genetic heterogeneity (where the same phenotype may be produced by different genes) and with reduced penetrance (where individuals with predisposing genes may not always have epilepsy, or even the EEG abnormalities associated with it). The inheritance pattern may not be clear-cut, and environmental and other influences may affect the expression of the epilepsy phenotype, often in an age-related pattern, which complicates the analysis of linkage data. It is possible to utilize computer programs that take these factors into account, but it is the programmers who must decide the age-related penetrance of the type of epilepsy under study and the type of inheritance, and they must be careful to validate these assumptions as fully as possible (Leppert, 1990; Elston, 1991).

Linkage analysis using 'random' markers

There are three types of epilepsy in which single-gene inheritance has been established (or is likely) and the location of the gene responsible has been identified by linkage analysis.

Benign familial neonatal convulsions

This rare condition is inherited as an autosomal dominant trait; otherwise healthy neonates develop frequent generalized or focal seizures that usually remit after a few months leaving no neurological sequelae. This condition was found to be linked to loci on the long arm of chromosome 20 in several families (Leppert et al, 1989; Malafosse et al, 1992). However, in another study a minority of families, where the convulsions started after the second day of life and always remitted by 2 months, did not appear to show linkage of the disease to the same region of the genome, indicating genetic heterogeneity (Ryan et al, 1991). In this study the family that did show linkage to chromosome 20 had a significant risk of subsequent epilepsy in affected individuals.

Juvenile myoclonic epilepsy (JME)

This is a common generalized epilepsy with a strong genetic component, although the pattern of inheritance is not always clear. Myoclonic seizures characteristically develop in otherwise normal adolescents on awakening, associated with generalized tonic–clonic seizures and absences, and are usually non-progressive, although long-term medication may be required. In parents and siblings of probands there is a high incidence of epileptic seizures of various types (absence, myoclonic or generalized tonic–clonic) and a higher incidence of EEG abnormalities (4–6-Hz multi-spike wave complexes) (Doose and Baier, 1987b). The inheritance has been described as polygenic. However, in certain families linkage to chromosome 6p21.3 marker loci (the HLA region) has been demonstrated, using both the recessive and dominant models and scoring individuals with only the EEG abnormalities as affected (Greenberg et al, 1988). In this study, linkage did not hold if only epileptic individuals were scored as affected. Another study, however, demonstrated linkage to this region of chromosome 6p under a dominant model of inheritance, but most convincingly if individuals with seizures were scored as affected (Weissbecker et al, 1991).

Recently, linkage analysis has been undertaken in a third set of 25 families composed of patients with JME who had at least one first-degree relative with idiopathic generalized epilepsy. The families were ascertained from the UK and Sweden. No significant evidence in favour of linkage was obtained at any locus under any of the models tested. These observations are in marked contrast to those previously published and suggest that either the previous evidence of linkage is spurious or that genetic heterogeneity exists within this epilepsy phenotype (Whitehouse et al, 1993).

Progressive myoclonus epilepsy of Unverricht–Lundborg

This is a rare autosomal recessive type of progressive epilepsy with an onset of seizures between 6 and 15 years of age associated with neurological deterioration (Norio and Koskiniemi, 1979). Linkage studies in Finland, where the disease is common, have established linkage to marker loci on chromosome 21q22 (Lehesjoki et al, 1991).

Candidate genes

Genes considered include those encoding proteins involved in inhibition of neuronal activity, inactivation of neurotransmitters, regulation of calcium binding and transport of ions across excitable membranes. Biochemical abnormalities have been identified in animals prone to seizures: γ-amino-butyric acid (GABA) receptors are abnormally increased in the substantia nigra and periventricular grey matter of mongolian gerbils, GABA-ergic or glutamate decarboxylase (GAD)-containing neurones and nerve terminals are abnormally increased in the hippocampus of mongolian gerbils and the inferior colliculi of epilepsy-prone mice (sound induced). Absence-like seizures may be induced by γ-hydroxybutyric acid and opiate receptor agonists, the antiepileptic drug ethosuximide blocks T-type calcium channels in thalamic cells, and noradrenaline terminals are increased in cerebral cortices of tottering mice with spike-wave seizures (Delgado-Escueta et al, 1986). Defects in GABA A-mediated inhibition may be associated with epilepsy: seizures may result from inhibition of GABA A synthesis or GABA A receptor blockade, and certain anticonvulsants react with these receptors (Gardiner, 1990). There are several subunits of the GABA A receptor and the genes for these are being located (chromosomes 4, 5 and X). Other candidate genes, many of which have been mapped and cloned, include the nerve growth factor b-subunit on chromosome 1, the Na/K ATPases on chromosomes 1, 13 and 19, the G proteins (chromosomes 1, 3 and 20), the sodium channel (chromosome 2), somatostatin (chromosome 3), certain proto-oncogenes and monoamine oxidase A (chromosome X) (Delgado-Escueta et al, 1991). Such genes could be candidates for epilepsy susceptibility genes, and linkage between types of epilepsy and polymorphisms at or close to these gene loci may be sought.

RISK ASSESSMENT FOR GENETIC COUNSELLING

Because of the heterogeneity of epilepsy, the establishment of an accurate diagnosis is imperative for genetic counselling. As with other branches of medicine the first step is to obtain a good clinical history. In suspected epilepsy it is especially important to obtain a good eye-witness account of the attacks and this may involve taking time to interview not just the parents but school staff, friends or other individuals. Episodes of disturbed consciousness in childhood are not always epileptic. Children suffer with febrile convulsions, faints, breath-holding attacks and reflex anoxic seizures. A history from the child may help in the differential: was there an aura or postictal confusion? Rarely, loss of consciousness may be the result of a cardiac conduction abnormality.

The age of onset of seizures may be important diagnostically. In the case of neonatal seizures the cause in the first 24 h of life may be pyridoxine dependency; between 24 and 72 h, glycine encephalopathy or glycogen synthase deficiency; between 72 h and 1 week, methylmalonic or propionic acidaemia (Fenichel, 1993). It is important to take a developmental history: is development normal, has it always been delayed, has it slowed or stopped with the onset of seizures, is there evidence of dementia? Remember that development starts in utero: was the pregnancy normal? Were there problems associated with the birth? (These, like relatively trivial head injury, may sometimes be irrelevant.)

Obtaining a good family history may be particularly difficult because of the stigma associated with the diagnosis of epilepsy in some people's minds. The correct diagnosis may not have been made in relatives or they may deliberately have concealed attacks from doctors.

The clinical examination should include a search for the cutaneous signs of inherited conditions that are associated with epilepsy: neurofibromatosis, tuberous sclerosis, incontinentia pigmenti, hypomelanosis of Ito, for example. There may be other physical findings: storage diseases may manifest coarse features, hepatosplenomegaly and/or cardiomegaly; ataxia and loss of hearing or vision may occur in some monogenic conditions.

On the basis of the clinical history or of abnormal findings on clinical examination specific diagnostic tests may be indicated (a full discussion of these is beyond the scope of this chapter). It certainly seems appropriate to perform one or more EEGs (possibly including a sleep study) in the proband in order to make an accurate seizure diagnosis. It may be appropriate to arrange EEG studies in relatives. A Wood's light examination of the proband and relatives may be indicated if tuberous sclerosis is suspected. Radiography, computed tomography and magnetic resonance imaging may complement the other findings.

Empiric risks

If a specific diagnosis can be made, it may be possible to give accurate genetic counselling. However, in the majority of children with epilepsy no such diagnosis will be made. Under these circumstances empiric risks can be given, based on the sort of family studies discussed above.

Sibling risks

Anderson et al (1990) have summarized some of the general conclusions: when the proband develops idiopathic epilepsy before 15 years of age, the cumulative risk to age 40 years for siblings is 3–5%, compared with 1–2% for the general population. When more detailed information is available (Anderson and Hauser, 1990), the sibling risks for epilepsy become: (a) 2–3% if the proband has partial seizures, or if the seizure onset in the proband is after the age of 25 years; (b) 5–6% when the proband has absence or generalized tonic–clonic seizures, and also a generalized spike and wave EEG; (c) 8% when (in addition to the preceding combination) the proband's EEG also shows a photoparoxysmal response and/or multifocal spikes; (d) 8% when both the proband and one parent have primary generalized seizures (10–12% when either or both have a generalized spike and wave EEG); and (e) 12–15% for those tested siblings with a generalized spike and wave EEG pattern when the proband has a similar pattern.

Risks in offspring

According to Beck-Mannagetta et al (1989) there is an overall risk of epilepsy in offspring of epileptic patients of between 3% and 4%. This risk is 3–4 times that in the general population, based on the cumulative incidence of 1.1% by the age of 25 years ascertained from the population of Rochester, Minnesota (Hauser and Kurland, 1975). Tsuboi (1989) states that the general risk that an epileptic may have an epileptic child is between 1% and 5%. The risk is greatest if both parents have idiopathic primary generalized epilepsy and show spike–wave complex EEG abnormality. The risk is least—probably less than 1%—if the proband has symptomatic partial epilepsy of known (non-genetic) aetiology, if the marital partner's EEG is normal and if the family history is negative.

RISKS TO THE FETUS OF ANTIEPILEPTIC MEDICATION DURING PREGNANCY

Since the late 1960s it has been apparent that babies born to women taking anticonvulsant treatment have an increased risk of congenital malformation, particularly cleft lip and palate (Meadow, 1968; Kelley et al, 1984b). There is a two- to threefold increase in the congenital malformation rate, particularly of cleft lip and palate, growth retardation and impaired cognitive function in infants of women taking anticonvulsants in the first trimester. Phenytoin (hydantoin) is particularly implicated and a distinctive dysmorphic facial appearance has become recognized in the 'fetal hydantoin syndrome'. This includes prenatal-onset growth deficiency, developmental delay and cranio-facial abnormalities including trigonocephaly or microcephaly, a broad nasal bridge, epicanthic folds, ptosis, hypertelorism, short upturned nose and low-set malformed ears (Hanson and Smith, 1975; Kelley, 1984). Hypoplasia of the distal phalanges and nails may occur and the risk of such minor facial and digital features occurring in infants born to women taking phenytoin is about 30%, but major abnormalities probably occur in only 4–6% (Kelley et al, 1984a).

There may be specific features associated with certain drugs, although this is not certain as many women take more than one drug. A fetal trimethadione syndrome has been described, comprising developmental delay, urogenital and skeletal malformations with dysmorphic facial features including V-shaped eyebrows, epicanthus, palatal clefting, ear abnormalities and developmental delay (Zackai et al, 1975; Feldman et al, 1977). A separate fetal valproate syndrome is recognized, with a 2–10% risk of neural tube defects in exposed fetuses and characteristic facial features including epicanthic folds continuing inferiorly and laterally to form a crease under the orbit, flat nasal bridge, small upturned nose, long upper lip with shallow philtrum and thin upper vermilion border and downturned angles of the mouth. Psychomotor delay may be associated (DiLiberti et al, 1984). There may be an increased risk of fetal loss (Jager-Roman et al, 1986).

There is less information about other anticonvulsants and phenobarbitone may be less teratogenic than phenytoin, but the evidence is that all carry some risk of causing fetal malformation. This obviously creates a dilemma in the management of pregnant epileptic women who require medication since seizure frequency may increase in pregnancy and status epilepticus in pregnancy may have an adverse effect on the fetus, although conclusive evidence about this is lacking. Valproate is probably the most potent teratogen of the anti-convulsants and it may be advisable in some circumstances, in consultation with the obstetrician and the neurologist, to change the regimen in favour of carbamazepine before or early in the pregnancy (Baraitser, 1990). Antenatal screening with fetal ultrasonography may be offered, looking for spina bifida, facial clefting and cardiac malformations in particular (Brodie, 1990).

THE FUTURE

Clinicians must all now be aware of the dramatic impact that the 'new genetics' has had on research in medicine. This has already been felt in the study of the epilepsies, despite the difficulties resulting from the complexity of the subject. Progress depends on collaboration between clinicians and molecular biologists, since a correct diagnosis is of critical importance for accurate molecular studies. Correct diagnosis depends on a progressively more sophisticated classification of seizures and seizure syndromes. It is therefore important that clinicians keep up to date with the modifications that are being made to the existing schemes of classification.

The key to genetic research is the family study, however complicated the research techniques and however extensive the data analysis. The clinician provides the cornerstone of this area of research by identifying the families that deserve special attention. Anderson and colleagues (1991b) have suggested that clinicians should look for the following:

1. Families with more than one affected sibling.
2. Patients who are twins.
3. An X-linked recessive pattern of inheritance.
4. A maternal inheritance pattern.
5. Epileptic patients with chromosome anomalies.
6. A series of probands ascertained a generation ago. In age-dependent seizure syndromes this may be the only way to obtain good EEG recordings during the age of risk for two generations of a family.

It seems unlikely that a single mechanism will be found to explain all types of epilepsy. However, there may be a few common underlying mechanisms. There is evidence that epilepsy genes are situated on specific chromosomes in three types of epilepsy: benign familial neonatal convulsions (chromosome 20), juvenile myoclonic epilepsy (chromosome 6) and progressive myoclonus epilepsy of Unverricht–Lundborg (chromosome 21). The hope is that certain epilepsy genes will soon be cloned but, as pointed out by Delgado-Escueta and co-workers (1986), the molecular defect is difficult to identify. In their review they discuss the use of animal models of epilepsy to identify candidate genes for human studies. Gardiner (1990) has reservations about this approach, drawing attention to the vast number of genes expressed in the brain and our ignorance of the underlying pathophysiology of the epilepsies.

In the last 10 years, collaborative research has led to remarkable discoveries about the genetics of neurological disorders. Such collaborative work has already yielded much information about the genetics of the epilepsies and we can expect to see continuing progress.

SUMMARY

The epilepsies are difficult to study because they are a heterogeneous group of disorders, both clinically and genetically. However, the classification of seizure types and epilepsy syndromes has given clinicians the means to define more accurately the distinct subtypes of epilepsy.

Evidence that epilepsy is inherited has come from various sources. Epidemiological studies, particularly family studies, have shown that there is an increased genetic risk of epilepsy in some families, although the seizure phenotype does not correspond exactly in different members. Animal studies have provided evidence for the existence of epilepsy genes and have suggested mechanisms of seizure production.

Many monogenic disorders are associated with seizures and the clinician should consider both these and chromosomal defects. Other types of inheritance may be relevant: multifactorial inheritance, mitochondrial inheritance and genomic imprinting.

Molecular genetic techniques have been applied to the study of the epilepsies. There is evidence that single-gene inheritance occurs in three types of epilepsy: benign familial neonatal convulsions, juvenile myoclonic epilepsy and progressive myoclonus epilepsy of Unverricht–Lundborg. There is hope that the first epilepsy gene will soon be cloned.

Clinicians can contribute to research in this area by promoting good clinical practice; guidelines for this are discussed. Information is given for the empiric assessment of the genetic risk of epilepsy for siblings and offspring of affected cases. There is also a discussion of the risks to the fetus of anticonvulsant drugs taken by the mother during pregnancy.

REFERENCES

Anderman E (1982) Multifactorial inheritance of generalized and focal epilepsy. In Anderson VE, Hauser WA, Penry JK & Sing CF (eds) *Genetic Basis of the Epilepsies*, pp 355–374. New York: Raven Press.

Anderson VE & Hauser WA (1990) The genetics of epilepsy. In Dam M & Gram L (eds) *Comprehensive Epileptology*, pp 57–76. New York: Raven Press.

Anderson VE, Wilcox KL, Rich SS et al (1989) Twin studies in epilepsy. In Beck-Mannagetta G, Anderson VE, Doose H & Janz D (eds) *Genetics of the Epilepsies*, pp 145–155. Berlin: Springer.

Anderson VE, Hauser WA, Olafsson E & Rich SS (1990) Genetic aspects of the epilepsies. In Sillanpää M, Johansson SI, Blennow G & Dam M (eds) *Paediatric Epilepsy*, pp 37–56. London: Wrightson Biomedical.

Anderson VE, Hauser WA, Leppik IE et al (eds) (1991a) *Genetic Strategies in Epilepsy Research (Epilepsy Research Supplement 4)*. Amsterdam: Elsevier.

Anderson VE, Rich SS, Hauser WA & Wilcox KJ (1991b) Family studies of epilepsy. In Anderson VE, Hauser WA, Leppik IE et al (eds) *Genetic Strategies in Epilepsy Research (Epilepsy Research Supplement 4)*, pp 89–103. Amsterdam: Elsevier.

Baraitser M (1990) *The Genetics of Neurological Disorders. Oxford Monographs on Medical Genetics*, 2nd edn, pp 110–112. Oxford: Oxford University Press.

Beck-Mannagetta G, Janz D, Hoffmeister U et al (1989) Morbidity risk for seizures and epilepsy in offspring of patients with epilepsy. In Beck-Mannagetta G, Anderson VE, Doose H & Janz D (eds) *Genetics of the Epilepsies*, pp 119–126. Berlin: Springer.

Bird TD (1987) Genetic considerations in childhood epilepsy. *Epilepsia* **28 (supplement 1):** S71–S81.

Blandfort M, Tsuboi T & Vogel F (1987) Genetic counselling in the epilepsies. I. Genetic risks. *Human Genetics* **76:** 303–331.

Bray PF & Wiser WC (1965) Hereditary characteristics of familial temporo-central focal epilepsy. *Pediatrics* **36:** 207–211.

Brodie M (1990) Management of epilepsy during pregnancy and lactation. *Lancet* **336:** 426–427.

Carter CO (1969) Genetics of common disorders. *British Medical Bulletin* **25:** 52–57.

Christodoulou J, Hall RK, Menaham S et al (1988) A syndrome of epilepsy, dementia, and amelogenesis imperfecta: genetic and clinical features. *Journal of Medical Genetics* **25:** 827–830.

Clarke-Fraser F (1980) Evolution of a palatable multifactorial threshold model. *American Journal of Human Genetics* **32:** 796–813.

Commission on Classification and Terminology of the International League Against Epilepsy (1989) Proposal for revised classification of epilepsies and epileptic syndromes. *Epilepsia* **30:** 389–399.

Dalla Bernardina B, Sgro V, Fontana E et al (1992) Idiopathic partial epilepsies in children. In Roger J, Bureau M, Dravet Ch et al (eds) *Epileptic Syndromes in Infancy, Childhood and Adolescence*, 2nd edn, pp 173–188. London: John Libbey

Davies K (1992) Imprinting and splicing join together. *Nature* **360:** 492.

Delgado-Escueta AV, Ward AA Jr, Woodbury DM & Porter RJ (1986) New wave of research in the epilepsies. *Advances in Neurology* **44:** 3–55.

Delgado-Escueta AV, Greenberg DA, Weissbecker K et al (1991) The choice of epilepsy syndromes for genetic analysis. In Anderson VE, Hauser WA, Leppik IE et al (eds) *Genetic Strategies in Epilepsy Research (Epilepsy Research Supplement 4)*, pp 147–159. Amsterdam: Elsevier.

DeLorenzo RJ (1991) The challenging genetics of epilepsy. In Anderson VE, Hauser WA, Leppik IE et al (eds) *Genetic Strategies in Epilepsy Research (Epilepsy Research Supplement 4)*, pp 3–17. Amsterdam: Elsevier.

DiLiberti JH, Farndon PA, Dennis NR & Curry CJR (1984) The fetal valproate syndrome. *American Journal of Medical Genetics* **19:** 473–481.

DiMauro S, Ricci E, Hirano M & DeVivo DC (1991) Epilepsy in mitochondrial encephalo-myopathies. In Anderson VE, Hauser WA, Leppik IE et al (eds) *Genetic Strategies in Epilepsy Research (Epilepsy Research Supplement 4)*, pp 173–180. Amsterdam: Elsevier.

Doose H & Baier WK (1987a) Genetic factors in epilepsies with primary generalized minor seizures. *Neuropediatrics* **18 (supplement I):** 1–64.

Doose H & Baier WK (1987b) Epilepsy with primary generalised myoclonic–astatic seizures: a genetically determined disease. *European Journal of Paediatrics* **146:** 550–554.

Doose H & Baier WK (1991) A genetically determined basic mechanism in benign partial epilepsies and related non-convulsive conditions. In Anderson VE, Hauser WA, Leppik IE et al (eds) *Genetic Strategies in Epilepsy Research (Epilepsy Research Supplement 4)*, pp 113–118. Amsterdam: Elsevier.

Doose H, Gerken H, Horstman T & Volzke E (1973) Genetic factors in spike-wave absences. *Epilepsia* **14:** 57–75.

Elston RC (1991) Genetic analysis of multivariate traits. In Anderson VE, Hauser WA, Leppik IE et al (eds) *Genetic Strategies in Epilepsy Research (Epilepsy Research Supplement 4)*, pp 161–171. Amsterdam: Elsevier.

Emery AEH & Mueller RF (1992) *Elements of Medical Genetics*, 8th edn, pp 188–191. London: Churchill Livingstone.

Falconer MA, Serafetinides EA & Corsellis JAN (1964) Etiology and pathogenesis of temporal lobe epilepsy. *Archives of Neurology* **10:** 233–248.

Feldman GL, Weaver DD & Lovrein EW (1977) The fetal trimethadione syndrome. *American Journal of Diseases of Children* **131:** 1389–1392.

Fenichel GM (1993) Paroxysmal disorders. In *Clinical Pediatric Neurology. A Signs and Symptoms Approach*, 2nd edn, pp 1–43. Philadelphia: WB Saunders.

Francois J (1982) Metabolic tapetoretinal degenerations. *Survey of Ophthalmology* **26(6):** 292–333.

Gardiner RM (1990) Genes and epilepsy. *Journal of Medical Genetics* **27:** 537–544.

Greenberg DA, Delgado-Escueta AV, Widelitz BH et al (1988) Juvenile myoclonic epilepsy (JME) may be linked to the BF and HLA foci on human chromosome 6. *American Journal of Medical Genetics* **31:** 185–192.

de Grouchy J & Turleau C (1984) *Clinical Atlas of Human Chromosomes*, 2nd edn. London: John Wiley.

Guerrini R, Bureau M, Maltei M-G et al (1990) Trisomy 12p syndrome: a chromosomal disorder associated with generalised 3-Hz spike and wave discharges. *Epilepsia* **31**: 557–566.

Hall JG (1990) Genomic imprinting: review and relevance to human diseases. *American Journal of Human Genetics* **46**: 857–873.

Hanson JW & Smith DW (1975) The fetal hydantoin syndrome. *Journal of Pediatrics* **87**: 285–290.

Harding AE (1989) Ramsay Hunt syndrome, Unverricht–Lundberg disease, or what? *Movement Disorders* **4**: 18–19.

Hauser WA & Kurland LF (1975) The epidemiology of epilepsy in Rochester, Minnesota, 1935 through 1967. *Epilepsia* **21**: 399–412.

Hayden M (1981) *Huntington's Chorea.* Berlin: Springer.

Heijbel J, Blom S & Rasmuson M (1975) Benign epilepsy of childhood with centrotemporal EEG foci: a genetic study. *Epilepsia* **16**: 285–293.

Hodgson SV (1991) Genomic imprinting. *Developmental Medicine and Child Neurology* **33**: 552–556.

Hodgson SV & Maher ER (1993) *A Practical Guide to Human Cancer Genetics.* Cambridge: Cambridge University Press.

Holt IJ, Harding AE, Cooper JM et al (1989) Mitochondrial myopathies; clinical and biochemical features of 30 patients with major deletions of muscle mitochondrial DNA. *Annals of Neurology* **26**: 699–708.

Jager-Roman E, Deichl A, Jakob S et al (1986) Fetal growth, major malformations and minor anomalies in infants born to women receiving valproic acid. *Journal of Pediatrics* **108**: 997–1004.

Janz D, Christian W (1957) Impulsiv-petitnal. *Deutsch Zeitschrift Nervenheik* **176**: 346–386.

Kelley TE (1984) Teratogenicity of anticonvulsant drugs. I. Review of the literature. *American Journal of Medical Genetics* **19**: 413–434.

Kelley TE, Edwards P, Rein M et al (1984a) Teratogenicity of anticonvulsant drugs. II. A prospective study. *American Journal of Medical Genetics* **19**: 435–443.

Kelley TE, Rein M & Edwards P (1984b) Teratogenicity of anticonvulsant drugs. IV. The association of clefting and epilepsy. *American Journal of Medical Genetics* **19**: 451–458.

Kobyashi Y, Momoi MY, Tominaga K et al (1991) Respiration deficient cells are caused by a single point mutation in the mitochondrial tRNA Leu (UUR) gene in mitochondrial myopathy, encephalopathy, lactic acidosis and stroke-like episodes (MELAS). *American Journal of Human Genetics* **49**: 590–599.

Lehesjoki AE, Koskienemi M, Sistonen P et al (1991) Localisation of a gene for progressive myoclonus epilepsy to chromosome 21q22. *Proceedings of the National Academy of Sciences of the USA* **88**: 3696–3699.

Leppert MF (1990) Gene mapping and other tools for discovery. *Epilepsia* **31 (supplement 3):** S11–S18.

Leppert M, Anderson VE, Quattlebaum T et al (1989) Benign familial neonatal convulsions linked to genetic markers on chromosome 20. *Nature* **337**: 647–648.

Leviton A & Cowan LD (1982) Epidemiology of seizure disorders in children. *Neuroepidemiology* **1**: 40–83.

Malafosse A, Leboyer M, Dulac O et al (1992) Confirmation of linkage of benign familial neonatal convulsions to D20S19 and D20S20. *Human Genetics* **89**: 54–58.

Meadow SR (1968) Anticonvulsant drugs and congenital abnormalities. *Lancet* **ii**: 1296.

Meijers-Heijboer EJ, Sandkuijl LA, Brunner HG et al (1992) Linkage analysis with chromosome 15q11–13 markers shows genomic imprinting in familial Angelman syndrome. *Journal of Medical Genetics* **29**: 853–857.

Metrakos JD & Metrakos K (1960) Genetics of convulsive disorders. I: Introduction, problems, methods and baselines. *Neurology* **10**: 228–240.

Metrakos K & Metrakos JD (1961) Genetics of convulsive disorders. II: Genetic and electroencephalographic studies in centrencephalic epilepsy. *Neurology* **11**: 474–483.

Metrakos K & Metrakos JD (1974) Genetics of epilepsy. In Magnus O & Lorentz de Haas AM (eds) *Handbook of Clinical Neurology, vol. 15. The Epilepsies,* pp 426–439. Amsterdam: North Holland.

Noebels JL (1991) Mutational analysis of spike-wave epilepsy phenotypes. In Anderson VE, Hauser WA, Leppik IE et al (eds) *Genetic Strategies in Epilepsy Research (Epilepsy Research Supplement 4),* pp 201–212. Amsterdam: Elsevier.

Noebels JL (1992) Molecular genetics and epilepsy. In Pedley TA & Meldrum BS (eds) *Recent Advances in Epilepsy*, No. 5, pp 1–13. London: Churchill Livingstone.

Norio R & Koskiniemi M (1979) Progressive myoclonus epilepsy: genetic and nosological aspects with special reference to 107 Finnish patients. *Clinical Genetics* 15: 382–398.

Osborne JP (1988) Diagnosis of tuberous sclerosis. *Archives of Disease in Childhood* 63: 1423–1425.

Ottman R (1989) Genetics of the partial epilepsies: a review. *Epilepsia* 30: 107–111.

Ottman R, Hauser WA & Susser M (1985) Genetic and maternal influences on susceptibility to seizures. An analytic view. *American Journal of Epidemiology* 122: 923–939.

Ottman R, Annegers JF, Hauser WA & Kurland LT (1988) Higher risk of seizures in offspring of mothers than of fathers with epilepsy. *American Journal of Human Genetics* 43: 257–264.

Qiao X & Noebels JL (1991) Genetic and phenotypic heterogeneity of inherited spike-wave epilepsy: two mutant gene loci with independent cerebral excitability defects. *Brain Research* 555: 43–50.

Reik W (1988) Genomic imprinting: a possible mechanism for the parental effect of Huntington's chorea. *Journal of Medical Genetics* 25: 805–808.

Riccardi VM & Eichner JE (1986) *Neurofibromatosis: Phenotype, Natural History and Pathogenesis*. Baltimore: Johns Hopkins University Press.

Rise ML, Frankel WN, Coffin JM & Seyfried TN (1991) Genes for epilepsy mapped in the mouse. *Science* 253: 669–673.

Ryan SG, Wiznitzer M, Hollman C et al (1991) Benign familial neonatal convulsions: evidence for clinical and genetic heterogeneity. *Annals of Neurology* 29: 469–473.

Seyfried TN & Glaser GH (1985) A review of mouse mutants as genetic models of epilepsy. *Epilepsia* 26: 143–150.

Seyfried TN, Glaser GH, Yu RK & Palayoor ST (1986) Inherited convulsive disorders in mice. *Advances in Neurology* 44: 115–133.

Shoffner JM, Lott MT, Lezza AMS et al (1990) Myoclonic epilepsy and ragged red fibre disease (MERFF) is associated with a mitochondrial DNA tRNA Lys mutation. *Cell* 61: 931–937.

Shorvon S (1991) Epidemiological studies of epilepsy and their contribution to genetics. In Anderson VE, Hauser WA, Leppik IE et al (eds) *Genetic Strategies in Epilepsy Research (Epilepsy Research Supplement 4)*, pp 53–68. Amsterdam: Elsevier.

Tangye SR (1979) The EEG and incidence of epilepsy in Down's syndrome. *Journal of Mental Deficiency Research* 23: 17–24.

Tsuboi T (1989) Genetic risks in offspring of epileptic parents. In Beck-Mannagetta G, Anderson VE, Doose H & Janz D (eds) *Genetics of the Epilepsies*, pp 111–118. Berlin: Springer.

Tsuboi T & Christian W (1973) On the genetics of primary generalized epilepsy with sporadic myoclonias of impulsive petit mal type. *Humangenetik* 19: 155–182.

Tsuboi T & Endo E (1991) Genetic studies of febrile convulsions: analysis of twin and family data. In Anderson VE, Hauser WA, Leppik IE et al (eds) *Genetic Strategies in Epilepsy Research (Epilepsy Research Supplement 4)*, pp 119–128. Amsterdam: Elsevier.

Veal RM (1974) The prevalence of epilepsy amongst mongols related to age. *Journal of Mental Deficiency Research* 18: 99–106.

Verity CM & Golding J (1991) Risk of epilepsy after febrile convulsions: a national cohort study. *British Medical Journal* 303: 1373–1376.

Wagstaff J, Knoll JHM, Glatt KA et al (1992) Maternal but not paternal transmission of 15q11–13 linked nondeletion Angelman syndrome leads to phenotypic expression. *Nature Genetics* 1: 219–234.

Wallace DC (1989) Mitochondrial DNA mutations and neuromuscular disease. *Trends in Genetics* 5: 9–13.

Weissbecker KA, Durner M, Janz D et al (1991) Confirmation of linkage between juvenile myoclonic epilepsy locus and the HLA region of chromosome 6. *American Journal of Medical Genetics* 38: 32–36.

Whitehouse W & Gardiner M (1991) Molecular and genetic aspects of epilepsy. *Current Opinion in Neurology and Neurosurgery* 4: 903–907.

Whitehouse W, Rees M, Parker K et al (1993) *Linkage analysis of idiopathic generalised epilepsy and marker loci on chromosome 6p in families of patients with juvenile myoclonic epilepsy: exclusion data around HLA suggests genetic heterogeneity*. Meeting of the British Paediatric Neurology Association, London (abstract). Institute of Child Health, January.

Wienker TF, von Reutern GM & Ropers HH (1979) Progressive myoclonus epilepsy: a variant with probable X-linked inheritance. *Human Genetics* **49:** 83–89.

Wolf P (1991) The phenotype: seizures and epilepsy syndromes. In Anderson VE, Hauser WA, Leppik IE et al (eds) *Genetic Strategies in Epilepsy Research (Epilepsy Research Supplement 4)*, pp 19–29. Amsterdam: Elsevier.

Zackai EH, Mellman WJ, Neiderer B & Hanson JW (1975) The fetal trimethadione syndrome. *Journal of Pediatrics* **87:** 280–284.

4

Paediatric epilepsy in developing countries

HASAN AZIZ
ROBERT C. WOODY

A child or adolescent with epilepsy in a developing country tends to present more challenging problems than his or her counterpart in a developed nation for reasons that include: (1) inadequate personnel and expertise in clinical neurosciences; (2) unpredictable supplies or unavailability of antiepileptic drugs; (3) poor patient compliance (due to inadequate education, different perceptions of illness and culturally determined treatment seeking behaviour); (4) reliance on non-standard systems of health care (herbal, homoeopathic etc.); (5) low priority given to epilepsy in the presence of other pressing national needs; and (6) poor communication and transportation facilities from rural areas to secondary and tertiary care centres.

Due to social perceptions of epilepsy, a child from Latin America, Africa or Asia is more likely to face isolation and discrimination than a child in a developed country. Epilepsy engenders isolation and discrimination unlike any other disease, than perhaps acquired immune deficiency syndrome (AIDS) today or leprosy in the past.

If there are solutions to the special problems facing the child with epilepsy in developing, low-technology societies, they are unlikely to be found by imitation of 'Western' medical models. In 1993, Lewis Thomas wrote:

> 'Let us assume that, in a flight of imagination, an economic state of affairs in which it is financially possible for richer countries to export replicas of their entire technology of medical care to the poor nations. This would involve, I suppose, prefabricated versions of Massachusetts General Hospital . . . installed in every city of middle Africa, Asia and South America . . . and money to sustain these enterprises for, at the least, a period of 25 years. I believe the net effect would be zero, or something less than zero. The affluent would save the airfares to fly them to hospitals in London or New York, but the masses of people . . . would be entirely unaffected, or perhaps even adversely affected, because of the investment of all available funds on technologies totally inappropriate to their health problems.'

The challenge for health-care workers in developing countries is to *adapt*, not *adopt*, Western medical practice. Epilepsy provides an excellent example.

A thorough review of the topic of epilepsy in developing countries was written by Shorvon and Farmer in 1988.

Baillière's Clinical Paediatrics—
Vol. 2, No. 3, August 1994
ISBN 0–7020–1862–7

507

FACTORS THAT DISTINGUISH DEVELOPED AND DEVELOPING COUNTRIES

It is important to recognize that the 'developing world' represents a large, heterogeneous group of nations and cultures. Any attempt to generalize about them creates major misconceptions. Characteristics that broadly apply, however, have been well described (Mausner and Kramer, 1985). Factors that particularly influence the outlook and care of children with seizure disorders in developing countries include:

1. A high crude birth rate (e.g. 35–50 per 1000 population) resulting in a large percentage of the population being under 15 years of age.
2. A high infant mortality rate (e.g. 50–180 deaths of infants under 1 year of age per 1000 live births. Not only deaths, but also excessive morbidity (such as congenital, genetic and acquired neurological disease) will occur. In developing nations, the postnatal component (death in infants older than 28 days but aged less than 1 year) of the infant mortality rate is of greatest importance.
3. A high crude death rate (e.g. 25 deaths per 1000 population) and high age-specific death rates in the very young.
4. Low literacy rates, especially among women and in rural populations.
5. Prejudice that favours male over female infants and children.
6. Inherent inferior roles and human rights for women, including opportunities for contraception, education and economic independence.
7. A low family per capita income, especially in rural areas.
8. A low physician to population ratio (e.g. one physician per 10 000 population).
9. Concentration of medical services in large cites with relatively few services in rural areas.
10. Poor levels of preventive health-care services and, increasingly, a desire to 'leapfrog' to status-rich tertiary health-care services.
11. Poor organization of basic health-care logistics such as pharmaceutical supply, requisition and distribution.
12. Poorly developed nursing and auxiliary health therapeutic services (laboratory services, physical therapy, social services etc.).
13. Considerable disease caused by trauma, infection and genetic causes; 'diseases of affluence' (arteriosclerosis, obesity and diabetes mellitus, tobacco-related diseases etc.) only now emerging as major problems for the future.
14. A bulky bureaucracy, often left over from colonial rule, impeding all aspects of health-care delivery.
15. A lack of national health schemes result in affluent or well-positioned individuals having the best available health care.

While an individual developing nation may be spared some of these traits, many nations' health-care systems suffer from all of them. Each characteristic directly affects the prevention, diagnosis and treatment of epilepsy and the psychosocial adjustment of children with epilepsy.

EPIDEMIOLOGY OF EPILEPSY IN DEVELOPING COUNTRIES

Reliable studies of the epidemiology of epilepsy in developing countries are starting to be published; research in this field is relatively new. Osuntokun (1978) could find only 20 reports that described epilepsy in Africans in the years 1957–1977. In 1987, Schoenberg emphasized the need for co-ordinated and thoughtful study of the neuroepidemiology of epilepsy in developing countries.

Particular attention should be paid to the difficulties of conducting epidemiological studies in developing nations. A major problem in generating incidence and prevalence data on epilepsy revolves around difficulties in ascertaining cases, classifying specific subgroups of patients and accurately measuring the denominators (populations) under study.

The reported incidence (number of new cases in a population in a specified period of time) of epilepsy in developing countries ranges widely from about 11 to 134 cases per 100 000 population, typically 20–70 cases per 100 000 (Shorvon and Farmer, 1988). The prevalence (total number of old and new cases in a population at a given time, or during a given period) usually ranges between 1.5 and 31 per 1000, usually falling between 4 and 10 cases per 1000 (Shorvon and Farmer, 1988). Generally it has been assumed that epilepsy is more common in developing than developed countries, but data to support this assumption are few.

A critical need is the development of techniques of data collection that are practical for societies with a low literacy rate. The creation of questionnaires with a high sensitivity, specificity and predictive value to screen for epilepsy in populations is of paramount importance. Similarly, validation of key informant techniques, surveys of pharmacy distribution of antiepileptic drugs and other indirect techniques of assessing the numbers of patients with seizures in a community require further study. Investigations that might serve as models for epidemiological studies of epilepsy in the developing world include work by Placencia et al (1992) in Ecuador, in which a cross-sectional study using a screening questionnaire was followed by a longitudinal study of a sample of patients undergoing therapy by a multi-disciplinary team. Feksi and Gatiti (1991) reported a study of 302 Kenyan patients with epilepsy identified by the key informant method, and compared this method to the random cluster sample method (Kaamugisha and Feksi, 1988). Osuntokun et al (1987a,b) used a door-to-door survey with a standardized questionnaire and simplified neurological examination conducted by primary health-care workers to detect epilepsy in a Nigerian village.

Specific social factors may need to be considered in many societies before accurate data can be gathered. For example, in many Muslim communities males outside the immediate family are denied access to women in the home. Therefore, house-to-house surveys are possible only if female surveyors are employed. Telephone surveys, so commonly performed in Western countries, are of no practical use in developing countries. A prejudice against female offspring may predetermine which sex of child is seen for medical attention of epilepsy, creating a sex bias in hospital-based studies. Misconceptions and fears about epilepsy by some of the population may lead the interviewer significantly to underestimate its prevalence in some communities.

CAUSES OF EPILEPSY IN DEVELOPING COUNTRIES

The aetiology of epilepsy has been the subject of many hospital-based studies, but selection bias introduced in these studies distorts the true portrayal of causes. Most reported population-based surveys of epilepsy from developing countries lack an in-depth study of risk factors because of limited access to investigative facilities.

The causes of epilepsy are similar in all developing countries. They can be broadly classified into genetic, malformations, perinatal (trauma, metabolic and hypoxic–ischaemic encephalopathy), infectious, vascular, toxic, postnatal, metabolic, nutritional and neurodegenerative. The overall frequency ratio of causes varies among populations, but certain causes that occur more often in developing countries will be discussed.

In most cases of epilepsy in developing countries a definite cause for the seizures cannot be proven; only tentative causes are offered. The overall frequency of identifiable cases worldwide varies from 17 to 45% in population-based studies (Hauser and Kurland, 1975; Goodridge and Shorvon, 1983; Li et al, 1985; Haerer et al, 1986; Srindharan et al, 1986; A. Guvener, personal communication, 1989). This wide variation is the result of both real factors and variation in case ascertainment among populations.

In developing countries, perinatal events, certain bacterial, viral and parasitic infections, and trauma are more common identifiable causes of seizures than in developed countries. Cranial trauma and hypoxic–ischaemic encephalopathy may be more common because of poorer ante-natal and immediate perinatal care. The extent of this problem is illustrated in a report from Saudia Arabia in which perinatal encephalopathy was reported in 40% of children with epilepsy (Al Rajeh et al, 1990). However, between 2 and 3% of cases of epilepsy in India and Nigeria were ascribed to perinatal events (Mani, 1987; Osunkotun et al, 1987a,b). Unfortunately these studies cannot be compared because of age-selection bias and differences in case ascertainment. Careful examination of the perinatal history is needed before events in this period can be accepted as causative of later epilepsy.

CNS infections, including meningoencephalitis, extra-axial suppurative infection and brain abscess, appear to be more common in developing countries because of poorer personal and community hygiene, greater family size, failure to make an early or correct diagnosis, inadequate health education, and inappropriate or outdated therapy. Cultural practices (bathing, diet, religious rituals etc.) may predispose infants and children to infectious and other environmental agents that cause epilepsy. Again, case selection and ascertainment bias make comparisons among studies from different countries difficult.

CNS tubercular granulomata appear to be uncommon even in developing countries, but in those patients who develop them, reported seizure rates are: 42.8% in Saudia Arabia (Bahemuka and Murungi, 1989) and 37.6% in India (Gulati et al, 1991).

Subacute sclerosing panencephalitis (SSPE) is much more common in the Middle East than in the West (Haddad et al, 1977). This preventable cause of myoclonic seizures presents with myoclonus or progressively worsening dementia, leading to death. Prior immunization with measles vaccine seems to prevent the occurrence of SSPE.

Parasitic infections of the CNS are a significant problem in developing countries. Neurocysticercosis is the result of the endemic presence of *Taenia* infestation in much of Africa, Asia and South America (Alarcon and Olivares, 1975; Gadjusek, 1978; Davis, 1983). Cysticercosis in Brazil has been reported in 13–27% of patients with epilepsy (Arruda, 1991), in Togo 38.7% (Dumas et al, 1989), in South African blacks 38% (Dancy et al, 1992) and in India 15.8% (Gulati et al, 1991). The Middle East is relatively free of both *Taenia saginatum* and *solium* infection, probably for cultural dietary reasons.

Seizures are also a common manifestation of acquired or congenital infection with *Toxoplasma gondii*. This organism is an opportunistic pathogen in patients with human immunodeficiency virus (HIV) infection (Bartolomei et al, 1991). A number of other parasitic or protozoan diseases may also cause seizures: schistosomiasis (Scrimgeour and Gadjusek, 1985), paragonimiasis (Chang et al, 1958), hydatidosis (Arseni and Marinescu, 1974), sparganosis (Fan and Pezeshkpour, 1986), toxocariasis (Elliot et al, 1985) and ascariasis (Dada, 1970). In areas of high malaria prevalence, seizures may often occur in children because of recurrent high fever or CNS malarial infection.

Even in developing countries, computed tomography (CT) is now commonly used to detect previously unrecognized radiographic correlates of epilepsy. Small isolated enhancing lesions of the brain have been reported frequently in patients from developing countries (Chandy et al, 1991). There has been considerable debate as to whether or not these lesions are tubercular or parasitic. Chandy and co-workers, in India, suggested that cysticercosis was the most common cause of these CT lesions. Caution in needed when interpreting supposed therapeutic success in this condition, since spontaneous disappearance may occur without therapeutic intervention.

HIV infection, a phenomenon increasingly found in developing countries of Africa, Latin America and Asia, may produce seizures as its first clinical symptom in about one third of patients (Bartolomei et al, 1991). Generalized seizures occur more often than partial ones. Primary HIV infection or secondary toxoplasmosis, progressive leukoencephalopathy, cytomegalovirus or other causes of meningoencephalitis may cause seizures.

A few neurodegenerative diseases, predominantly characterized by seizures, occur in developing countries. SSPE most commonly occurs in children who failed to receive measles immunization, allowing them to acquire the natural infection. 'See-ee' is an epileptic condition reported from both Tanzania (Jilek and Jilek-Aall, 1977) and the Grand Basa country in Liberia

(Goudsmit et al, 1983). The precise cause of this condition is unknown, but viral and local environmental factors may both contribute. In a study of 4436 members of a clan in Grand Basa County with 'see-ee', 123 cases of epilepsy were found; 38% of these cases were precipitated by a CNS infection and 53% of patients had a positive family history of similar seizures. The sex ratio was equal and the age of onset was usually 9–12 years. The disease appears to have been introduced into the community about 1950.

Another epileptic disorder peculiar to developing countries is 'hot-water epilepsy', a reflex epilepsy reported frequently from India. Hot bath-water poured repeatedly over the heads of children and adolescents may result in simple or complex partial seizures associated with intensely pleasurable feelings. Hot-water epilepsy is common, occurring more often in Muslims than in others in India (Mani et al, 1975). Gururaj and Satishchandra (1992) reported it in males more often than females (3.6:1), with 89% of patients having between one and four attacks per month. About 25% of patients had a past history of febrile seizures.

Head trauma is a major cause of epilepsy in developing countries. Motor vehicle and pedestrian accidents, falls and occupational injuries (even among young working children) are all excessively common in developing countries, predisposing the child to post-traumatic epilepsy.

Consanguinity is a common social practice in many areas of the developing world, especially in the Middle East, India and the Far East. Al Rajeh et al (1990) reported that 53% of parents of children with epilepsy were related by blood. However, the role of consanguinity as a cause of epilepsy is questionable. A large hospital-based study of 4463 seizure patients in Pakistan found no difference in the consanguinity rates of the parents of patients and those in the general population, or the rates in patients with primary seizures and those with secondary generalized seizures (Aziz et al, 1991a). Since only generalized epilepsies are thought to have a genetic basis, it is not surprising that consanguinity does not play a major role in the prevalence of epilepsy. Genetic aspects of this problem are discussed by Hodgson and Verity in Chapter 3.

Epilepsy has been reported to be more common in lower socio-economic groups. Two Nigerian population-based surveys using identical study designs found a seizure prevalence of 37 per 1000 in a poor village and 5.3 per 1000 in a higher socio-economic area 20 km away (Osuntokun et al, 1987a,b). The role of socio-economic factors in epilepsy is complex and perhaps relates indirectly through the effects of other health problems.

PERCEPTIONS OF EPILEPSY IN DEVELOPING COUNTRIES

In developing countries, the perception of epilepsy is still shrouded in myth, superstition and resignation to 'God's will'. References to black magic and evil spirits are often made by the families of seizure patients (Aziz et al, 1991b; A. Guvener, personal communication 1989). Many patients and families visit a community spiritual healer while receiving 'Western' medical care. Ten per cent of patients in Pakistan and 50% of those in Turkey believe that epilepsy is a non-medical problem. Many of these patients only took home remedies or consulted traditional healers (Aziz et al, 1991b; A. Guvener, personal communication 1989). In some areas of Zambia, seizure patients are the 'specialty' of traditional healers, thus blocking the inroads of Western medical care (B. Voetberg, personal communication 1991).

Despite these problems, an extensive survey of 8600 Mexicans recently described a high level of accurate understanding of the causes, treatment and psychosocial potential of seizure patients (Felipe et al, 1991).

CLASSIFICATION OF EPILEPSY

Epileptic seizures may be classified by clinical seizure type, aetiology, age of onset or the results of investigations. Each classification system has its merits and problems, especially when applied to developing countries. Comprehensive classification systems have been sequentially proposed by the International League Against Epilepsy (ILAE), most recently in 1981 and 1989. In this system, both clinical and EEG data are taken into account. Details of this classification are reviewed in Chapter 2.

Physicians working in developing nations where classification is based primarily on clinical phenomena still follow simpler divisions of major and minor, or general or focal epilepsies. Since current international neuro-logical literature now follows the ILAE classification individual medical practice often leads to communication difficulties when it comes to estab-lishing epidemiological databases. This seemingly simple problem is a major obstacle to therapy, logistical organization, prevention and education regarding epilepsy in developing countries. Hence there is a need to develop a widely accepted classification that is clearly understood and adopted by all neurological practitioners.

DIAGNOSIS OF EPILEPSY IN DEVELOPING COUNTRIES

The diagnosis of epilepsy should be clinical with maximum emphasis placed on eye-witness information. Investigations should be limited to those that are diagnostically or therapeutically necessary. Physician thresholds for deciding on studies vary widely from country to country, and will necessarily vary depending on the financial well-being of the family and the availability of financial support offered by the government or other sources. Medical personnel must be educated about the cost–effectiveness of diagnostic pro-cedures, especially as the costs of medical tests may mean that a family will not have income for food, housing or other essential needs. Unnecessary 'academic' investigations may have adverse effects: high cost to the family, and the generation of inappropriate fears and expectations.

For seizures of new onset, relevant investigations may be necessary. Especially in areas of endemic infections or toxic exposure, medical person-nel must be taught to focus on these factors when ordering investigations. Since there is often a long delay in receiving the results of studies, simple therapy should be started whilst awaiting confirmatory results. Convincing patients to return to clinic for the results is often difficult, and this problem must be overcome by family education that focuses on the roles of the family and the physician.

INDICATIONS FOR SPECIALIZED INVESTIGATIONS

The scarcity of local human and financial resources makes it necessary to refer seizure patients judiciously, and then to limit the number of neurodiagnostic investigations. Most children with epilepsy do not require special investigations; many do not require an EEG. In remote areas, an adequate basic clinical examination and thoughtful history by a suitably trained physician or community health worker is sufficient in most cases for diagnosis, allaying parental fear of severe underlying intracranial pathology and avoiding unnecessary expense. A few patients need neurodiagnostic investigations to exclude serious pathology (tumour, arteriovenous malformations etc.); these children may need specialized neurological expertise. In areas with minimal neurodiagnostic facilities, it may be difficult to select these few patients from the many hundreds or thousands of children with seizure disorders. The following commonsense guidelines, learned from our extensive experience in making such decisions in developing countries, may be helpful:

1. Focal seizures, especially if persistent, suggest an underlying focal pathology that needs investigation.
2. Fixed or progressive neurological deficits or increased intracranial pressure need to be explained.
3. A history of postictal (Todd's) paralysis lasting more than 6 h may suggest new and serious underlying focal disease.
4. Medically intractable seizures are a special problem, requiring referral.
5. Convulsions associated with febrile illnesses (which do not meet the criteria for febrile seizures) are often serious and may require neurosurgical intervention.

JUDICIOUS USE OF NEURODIAGNOSTIC PROCEDURES

As described above, the main emphasis in evaluating a child with seizures should always be on a thoughtful clinical history and physical examination. Neurodiagnostic studies are never a substitute for clinical appraisal. While neurophysiological and neuroradiological equipment is now available for purchase in nearly every nation, few developing countries can afford their liberal purchase and use, as other health priorities justifiably come first. Investigation should be limited to those tests that help pragmatically in the management of epilepsy. Relevant haematological, biochemical, metabolic and microbiological studies are well justified in many cases. Cerebrospinal fluid analysis should nearly always be possible, even in refugee camps. When used in cases of suspected intracranial infection, these studies have a high positive predictive value and are of great clinical worth, besides being economically feasible.

Neurophysiological studies (routine EEG, ambulatory EEG, video-EEG, sphenoidal EEG etc.) have a place in specialized epilepsy centres. Many physicians mistakenly believe that EEGs can confirm the presence or absence of epilepsy; this tendency should be actively discouraged by neurologists. Often, both the physician and technician have very limited training in performing and interpreting EEGs, and the quality of tracings is poor. An EEG can be helpful, but in most cases the history accurately provides the diagnosis and suggests first-line drug treatment. About 35% of seizure patients have an abnormal interictal EEG (Ajmone-Marsan and Zivin, 1970) and even in developed countries the basis of diagnosis in 65% of cases remains clinical. In developing countries, the EEG should be limited to certain secondary or tertiary care centres and restricted to patients who present with diagnostically difficult cases, drug-resistent epilepsy or those who might require surgical intervention.

The value of neuroimaging studies (CT and magnetic resonance imaging (MRI)) cannot be denied when adequate resources are available. Most available CT studies of epilepsy patients have been performed on hospital-based series, producing a major selection bias. In one study of 256 children with epilepsy, abnormalities on CT were found in 33% (Yang et al, 1979). The proportion of abnormal scans was greater in those children with focal neurological findings, a history of simple partial seizures, focal EEG findings and neonatal seizures. A much greater positive predictive value (70–80%) is seen in patients with focal neurological signs, a history of focal rather than generalized seizures, and focal EEG findings (Young et al, 1982).

In developing nations, the cost of these tools may represent a significant proportion of the national health-care budget. Only in light of other health-care priorities, especially those involving preventive care, can these neuro-diagnostic tools be justified. Analysis of neuroimaging cost: benefit is difficult to calculate in developing countries. The cost of a CT scan may exceed maintenance drug therapy for ten or more patients for 1 year, yet no data exist generally to quantify parameters such as Years of Productive Life Lost, individual and family psychosocial stress from epilepsy, etc.

In practice, patients in whom intracranial neoplasm and infection, resistant epilepsy and other specific neuropathology have been excluded clinically rarely require CT or MRI. Therefore, there is a limited (and even questionable) need for these imaging facilities, except in tertiary epilepsy referral centres, in a developing country.

TREATMENT OF EPILEPSY

Epilepsy in developing countries can be managed by health-care workers other than neurologists. The concept that the seizure patient must be treated by the specialist has no practical use in the developing world today, or in the foreseeable future. Although the number of neurologists in the developing world is increasing, it still is far below that needed to care for patients with neurological disease, especially epilepsy. In 1975, there were two neurologists in Syria for people of all ages, when the population was 8 000 000; today, there are about 30 neurologists for a population of nearly 13 000 000 but no paediatric neurologist (i.e. one neurologist for 433 000 population; compare this to the USA where there is 1 per 20 000 population). Shorvon and Farmer (1988) noted that, in 1977, Nigeria, with one quarter of all of Africa's population, there were only seven neurologists; in Ghana, with a population of 8 000 000, there are two neurologists. Neurologists must be prepared to work beside nurses, community health-care workers, 'health promoters' and even sociologists and anthropologists to deal with patients who may come from sociocultural backgrounds radically different from their own.

General medical practitioners and community health workers are highly likely to be required to care for children with epilepsy. Suitable training can prepare community health workers to recognize and begin treatment in many children (Meinardi, 1988; Feksi et al, 1991a,b; Shorvon et al, 1991). For community health workers to manage epilepsy correctly, they should be given simple guidelines in diagnosis, drug dosing, drug side-effect recognition and psychosocial counselling. After initial diagnosis and therapy, the care of the patient should be reviewed by a physician trained to care for epilepsy. Neurologists must routinely survey their work.

Medically trained personnel dealing with epilepsy must be prepared to work in tandem with local healers (Shorvon and Farmer, 1988; B. Voetberg, personal communication 1992). However, it must be emphasized that traditional advice may include persuading the parent to place the arm of a seizing child into fire, that the child's saliva will spread seizures, that the female child with epilepsy cannot safely marry later in life etc. Diplomacy and firmness, with an eye to the best long-term interests of the patient, are needed by the health-care worker.

THE DECISION TO START ANTIEPILEPTIC THERAPY

The decision process whether to start therapy for paediatric epilepsy in developing countries is similar to that in developed countries. Isolated or infrequent seizures do not usually require prophylactic therapy. More than two seizures in the previous year may justify therapy, but, even then, the family should be asked their opinion and be given accurate advice regarding the likely benefits and costs of seizures versus therapy. Treatment of infrequent seizures is likely to lead to non-compliance, as the family eventually recognizes the unfavourable cost : benefit relationship. Also, withdrawal seizures and status epilepticus may occur from sudden cessation of treatment, even when the seizure disorder has previously been only a minor problem. The treating health-care worker should remember that the chance of recurrence of a single seizure is about 20% (Hauser et al, 1982).

In developed countries the choice of antiepileptic medication usually depends on seizure type, but this principle may be difficult to employ in developing countries. Since neurophysiological studies may not be available, classification must rely on clinical history, which is dependent on the accuracy of the historian and the acumen of the clinician. Because of this, the choice of the 'correct antiepileptic drug' becomes somewhat meaningless. All four of the major drugs (phenobarbitone, phenytoin, carbamazepine and valproate) are approximately equally effective in the control of most types of seizure, although some may be better tolerated than others (Mattson et al, 1985; Shorvon et al, 1991). This statement probably applies to 95% of seizure patients. The profile of side-effects may be quite different for the four major antiepileptic drugs.

Relatively uncommon seizure types (particularly generalized forms such as myoclonus and absence) may require special therapeutic considerations. Absence (petit mal) responds best to sodium valproate (Editorial, 1988). Ethosuximide, the longer established therapy for absence, is rarely available in developing countries. Myoclonic seizures respond well to nitrazepam (Browne and Penry, 1973), clonazepam (Naito et al, 1987) and valproate. Nitrazepam tends to be less expensive and more readily available than other effective drugs.

Diazepam is an inexpensive and widely available antiepileptic drug in most developing countries. Its use is restricted to the intravenous treatment of status epilepticus and for prophylaxis of seizures (especially febrile seizures), with rectal use at home. It has no place in the management of chronic seizure disorders in children since it has little antiepileptic efficacy in this situation, is sedating, and may lead to habituation and physiological dependency following years of use.

The value of routine laboratory studies and drug concentration monitoring for antiepileptic drug therapy is a luxury that few developing nations can afford. Side-effects and overdosage can be detected clinically and the patient referred if necessary. Teaching auxiliary care personnel to handle such problems is a challenge and a necessity in developing countries.

All things considered, the overall condition of medical treatment of seizures in both adults and children in developing countries is poor. At any given time, only 6–20% of patients with active epilepsy are receiving drug therapy in developing countries (Shorvon and Farmer, 1988). In rural populations, the rate is likely to be even lower (Aziz, 1989). A useful method of estimating treatment status is use of the 'therapeutic gap' (Ellison et al, 1988). This is the number of patients with active epilepsy in a population (derived from the expected prevalence of epilepsy in the community) contrasted with those utilizing antiepileptic medication in the community (as determined by drug supply and sales). Ellison and co-workers have determined that the therapeutic gap in Pakistan, the Philippines and Ecuador ranges from 80 to 94%, i.e. only 6–20% of patients with active epilepsy at a given time are receiving drug therapy. The therapeutic gap in these countries is the same regardless of the cost of the drug prescribed; therefore the gap appears not to be a result of drug costs alone (Shorvon and Farmer, 1988).

In the developed world the cost of therapy can be taken as the cost of the medical visit, tests and medication prescription; in the developing world the cost is quite different. Owing to the lack of communication facilities, travel from long distances may be necessary to receive medical care. The patient and family will require housing and food for the visit. Income is lost. Often the family itself has to find a centre that will perform certain medical examinations, or find medications. Only cash is accepted as payment. In Syria, a CT scan now costs about 2000 Syrian lira and treatment with valproate for 1 month about 500 Syrian lira. The average worker's monthly salary is about 3000 lira.

Compounding these difficulties is the knowledge that epilepsy is a chronic disease. One visit will rarely produce a good result. The family often assumes that the doctor will write a curative prescription and that the patient's problem will be resolved. When cure does not occur, the family seeks other medical care. Instead, the patient and family must deal with the reality that a series of visits may be needed, at significant total cost to them. Regular scheduled visits, rather than emergency visits for acute seizures or drug toxicity, are preferable but often impractical. By providing a competent health-care worker near the family's home, a great community service can be done.

In considering surgical management of epilepsy in developing countries it should be appreciated that neurosurgical services are often inundated by patients with cranial trauma, tumours and intracranial infections. Intraoperative neurophysiological monitoring is a luxury that few developing nations possess or can afford. Appropriate and necessary neuro-psychological services are even more scarce. Despite these problems, successful epilepsy surgical units have been established in Argentina (Pomata et al, 1991) and Brazil (Rogazzo et al, 1991) and may serve as models for future units in developing countries. Only when surgical therapy for epilepsy is considered in the broadest context of the health-care needs of a developing country should investment be made in this direction.

TREATMENT FAILURES

Patient non-compliance with medical therapy is not unique to either epilepsy or the developing world. The reasons for non-compliance in developing countries has been little studied. Elechi (1991) reported that, among 45 adult seizure patients in Nigeria followed for two and a half years, there were 39 episodes of non-compliance among 19 patients. The main reasons given were the high costs or non-availability of antiepileptic drugs. Confusion over drug dosage and side-effects were other reasons for failure. Eighteen additional patients among the 45 studied failed to return for scheduled follow-up appointments in the seizure clinic. Overall, 82% of patients were either non-compliant or failed to keep appointments. Elechi (1991) recommended that seizure therapy be community based to maximize achievable compliance. Governments should also provide antiepileptic drugs at subsidized rates and provide logistical mechanisms to ensure a continuous supply of them at local pharmacies.

As a corollary to this work, Gatiti and Feksi (1991) reported a high success rate (85% 4-year patient compliance) and improved social integration into the community when Kenyan community health workers were trained to act as educators, supporters and links among the patient, doctor, family and community.

SPECIAL EPILEPSY CENTRES

In developing countries it is far more economical to have a few designated centres for the management of complex epilepsy cases than to have many medical departments with limited trained personnel and technological support. All too commonly, medical centres in a developing nations purchase state-of-the-art neurodiagnostic equipment, resulting in poor cost-efficiency. Such equipment often lies idle for lack of adequate support personnel. Often, the suppliers of such equipment are most interested in the sale and have little interest or ability to provide maintenance and service support. Some developed countries have been accused of 'dumping' out-of-date or used neurodiagnostic equipment into technologically under-developed nations.

Specialized epilepsy centres may prove to be useful in the diagnosis and management of paediatric epilepsy, provided that guidelines are established and adapted to local constraints. Efficient management, pharmaceutical supply, cost–benefit analysis of drugs and equipment, training, public education and study of local aetiological factors are all useful in avoiding waste of scarce resources.

The recent report of comprehensive epilepsy management in Kenya provides a valuable model for future health-care delivery (Feksi et al, 1991a,b). A public health-care perspective was adopted for the programme, including case identification, health-worker support, treatment protocols and levels of technology appropriate for rural Kenya. Review of medical records and key informants in the community were valuable in identifying people with epilepsy. Treatment with simple drug regimens was in the hands of primary health-care workers supervised by more experienced medical workers. While primary health-care workers accurately identified tonic–clonic seizures, they were less capable of recognizing complex partial seizures. Fifty-three per cent of patients became seizure free and a further 26% had a substantial decrease in the number of seizures at 6 months. Even those patients with long-standing untreated epilepsy had an acceptable response to therapy. Acceptable medical compliance indicates that primary health-care workers are able to monitor drug therapy for seizure patients in developing countries.

Albuquerque et al (1991) reported successful medical and psychosocial management of 37 Brazilian adult seizure patients by a multidisciplinary team approach.

COUNSELLING SEIZURE PATIENTS IN
DEVELOPING COUNTRIES

Whether in developed or developing countries, the degree of success in managing seizure patients is directly proportional to the amount of effort health-care workers put into educating patients and their families about the causes, therapy, prognosis and effects of epilepsy and antiepileptic drugs. In developing countries, additional factors usually not considered in 'Western' practice should also be mentioned. Local cultural perceptions of epilepsy, social stigmatization and patient expectations of physicians and local healers may affect treatment-seeking behaviour and compliance. In societies with poor literacy rates, epilepsy education may be difficult. Without education, the chances of compliance are slim. Simple explanations by community health workers may enhance compliance. Certainly, simple lessons such as the fact that the drugs do not cure, but only treat, epilepsy should be spelled out plainly. Understanding the need to maintain a continuous supply of drugs and to regularly take the medication should not be taken for granted in patients in any culture.

Genetic counselling is often sought by parents because of the perceived risk of genetic transmission. In Chapter 3 of this text, Hodgson and Verity deal in detail with the current basis and practice of genetic counselling in epilepsy. This topic is of particular sensitivity in developing countries since epilepsy may lead to stigmatization of an entire family and make marriage difficult or impossible, especially for females. Despite the need for information in this regard, few investigators have systematically studied the effective means of counselling patients in developing countries. As a guideline, the risk of recurrent non-febrile seizures in the offspring of one parent with seizures is 3.2–4.0% (Tsuboi and Endo, 1977; Annegers et al, 1982; Janz and Beck-Mannagetta, 1982), and approximately 10–13% if both parents have seizures (Metrakos and Metrakos, 1966; Annegers et al, 1982). Thus, in general, the risk is relatively small and should not deter marriage or childbearing. Despite this, epilepsy remains a major reason for excluding a female in consideration as a wife. Women in developing countries frequently hide their epilepsy from a prospective husband; divorce in many countries results when the husband realizes that the woman has seizures and has lied to him (S. Roumani, personal communication 1992).

THE PROGNOSIS OF CHILDHOOD EPILEPSY IN DEVELOPING COUNTRIES

Few studies have addressed the effectiveness of medical therapy of epilepsy in developing countries. Issues of epilepsy morbidity and mortality have also received little attention.

A series of recent reports has described the effectiveness of conventional medical therapy of epilepsy in the developing world. Jain and Maheshwari (1991) reported a prospective study, lasting for at least 3 years, of 306 seizure patients in India. Two thirds of patients treated with a single antiepileptic drug had 'adequate' results. Ismael (1990) documented results of phenobarbitone therapy on 117 Indonesian children with epilepsy (excluding those with infantile spasms). Good results were obtained in 62.4%, fair in 7.7%

and poor in 29.9%. Depending on seizure type, good results ranged from 72.6% in major motor seizures to 44% in complex partial seizures. In only two cases phenobarbitone was discontinued because of 'intolerable side-effects'. McFadyen et al (1990) described conventional antiepileptic drug therapy, accompanied by serum drug concentration monitoring, and a multidisciplinary team approach in a South African epilepsy clinic based at a large referral hospital. The proportion of patients with good control increased from 36 to 60%.

Feksi et al (1991a) described a primary-care therapy programme in Kenya. In this clinic treatment was provided largely by supervised primary health-care workers. Of 249 patients, 53% became seizure free and 26% had a substantial decrease in the number of seizures (greater than 50%).

Ogunniyi and Osuntokun (1991) described the results of antiepileptic drug therapy in 175 Nigerian adults; 126 received monotherapy and phenobarbitone was prescribed most commonly. Good to excellent seizure control was achieved in 67% of patients. Phenytoin and phenobarbitone were equally effective. Drug toxicity (mainly drowsiness and movement disorders) occurred in 61 patients. The investigators concluded that phenobarbitone should remain the major drug because of its low cost, availability and low level of side-effects.

From these studies, monotherapy with phenobarbitone seems most likely to provide the single most cost-effective therapy for epilepsy overall in developing countries. However, many neurologists in developed countries are hesitant to prescribe phenobarbitone as a first-line therapy because of its adverse side-effect profile. Noting the common, and at times severe, behavioural and cognitive effects of phenobarbitone in children, Shorvon and Farmer (1988) pointed out '. . . it is cynical to believe that these side-effects are of no importance in the less privileged developing countries. This is to put a geographic hierarchy on brain function, which is unacceptable.'

Injury associated with seizures is common in developing countries. In a study of 870 Sri Lankan seizure patients aged 5–85 years, 40% sustained an injury related to seizures, and 4% had had more than ten such injuries. Burns or scalds occurred in 62 patients and falls in a further 15 (Peiris and Senanayake, 1991).

Psychosocial adaptation to epilepsy in children is even more culturally dependent than medical therapy or morbidity and mortality from epilepsy. Schier et al (1991) pointed out that in tradition-bound societies epilepsy is seen as a major socially negative and handicapping condition. Issues of employment and transition from family life to independence are of major importance in both developed and developing nations (Kies et al, 1991; Parks-Trusz and Troxell, 1991). In the few studies of these problems in developing nations, emphasis has been placed on multidisciplinary therapy (including psychological, sociological and vocational evaluations) (Albuquerque at al, 1991) and community-centred care for epilepsy management (Gatiti and Feksi, 1991). Of particular importance are issues of epilepsy in adolescence (Avondet et al, 1991) and the impact of epilepsy on family life (Thompson and Upton, 1991).

PREVENTION OF EPILEPSY IN DEVELOPING COUNTRIES

Distinction must be made between primary, secondary and tertiary prevention. Primary prevention is the removal of risk factors or exposure from the individual at risk. Secondary prevention is detection of the disease at an early presymptomatic stage. Tertiary prevention is rehabilitation of the patient once an advanced disease state has been reached so that further handicap does not occur. In dealing with the child with epilepsy, the discussion should focus on primary and tertiary prevention, since secondary prevention is probably of little utility.

The opportunities to prevent epilepsy in children in developing countries are significant. Ogunniyi and Osuntokun (1991) examined risk factors for the development of epilepsy in Nigerians and found that two factors were associated with increased odds ratios: febrile seizures (OR = 11.0) and head trauma (OR = 13.0). A high primary childhood immunization rate was associated with a decreased risk of epilepsy, although this may have represented a marker of overall paediatric health and social care.

Although immunization against *Haemophilus influenzae* type b is now available worldwide, it is expensive and those under one require a series of immunizations. Despite this, in developed nations, *H. influenzae* infection, including meningoencephalitis, has decreased dramatically since introduction of the immunization. The incidence of *H. influenzae* meningoencephalitis declined in US Army children from 59 per 100 000 children in 1986 to 6 per 100 000 in 1991 (Broadhurst et al, 1993). The same could occur worldwide if national health budgets permitted widescale immunization against the bacterium.

The other most obvious preventive opportunity is the prevention of intracranial trauma, with particular regard to motor vehicles and pedestrians. Car seat belts are rarely installed in developing countries or used when they are available

Prevention of other infections, including tuberculosis, cysticercosis and echinococcosis, would be difficult but is possible. The elimination of measles and a reduction in pertussis is potentially achievable through high levels of infant immunization.

The prevention of perinatal brain injury from trauma and hypoxic ischaemic encephalopathy is more difficult, but is important. Secondary prevention by early neonatal screening for phenylketonuria and other inborn errors of metabolism is feasible but would probably contribute little to the overall control of epilepsy in developing countries.

On the other hand, tertiary prevention of psychosocial, educational and employment disability among children with epilepsy could be of great benefit and might be carried out inexpensively in developing countries. The seizure itself is usually of minor significance and of short duration; the psychosocial disability may be crippling and life-long. The development of educational and counselling services at local and regional levels in developing countries might be the wisest investment a country could make for these patients.

The decision to invest in prevention should rationally depend on the cost–benefit analysis of the situation. The cost of primary and tertiary prevention should be weighed against the costs of disease and disability. The cost of setting up and maintaining prevention may be quite high (assuming that populations are willing and capable of changing their behaviours in the first place). Benefits are difficult to measure in developing countries, where the birth rate is high and more than 50% of the population is under 15 years of age. Unemployment may be high, and social and rehabilitative services are few. Given these factors, what saving is made when epilepsy is prevented in one individual? Even in broadly preventing epilepsy in large numbers, what are the savings? In a society that is currently spending little or no money on the care of epilepsy, and in which individuals even if able bodied, have little opportunity to contribute substantially to society, the measurable savings will be minimal. Therefore, the cost–benefit analysis appears unfavourable. Only when the cost–benefit analysis in developing nations appears more favourable are national health care expenditures likely to be used to prevent epilepsy and its complications.

WORLD HEALTH ORGANIZATION RECOMMENDATIONS AND ESSENTIAL DRUG LISTS

In 1976, Gastaut and Osuntokun, writing for the WHO Collaborating Centers, noted: 'It has been pointed out that the developing countries should not imitate the industrialized ones, and they especially should avoid unnecessary expenditures on costly treatments . . . The developing countries would save a lot of money and assist epileptic patients by taking a different course and making available to their physicians a small number of products that are effective and harmless.'

The WHO, by setting international drug policies and by interacting with national governments, powerfully influences the choices of antiepileptic drugs available in local settings. The Essential Drug List is a comprehensive list of medications chosen because of their widespread availability on grounds of low cost, balanced efficacy and safety. In 1985, the WHO Second Report recommended that essential antiepileptic drugs should include diazepam, ethosuximide, phenobarbitone and phenytoin. Carbamazepine and valproate would be supplementary, for use in exceptional circumstances. In 1988, WHO Third Report recommended that carbamazepine and valproate be moved to the primary essential drug list, commented on the rectal use of diazepam and added a syrup formulation of ethosuximide for paediatric use.

Despite this evolution of recommendations, in practice phenobarbitone and phenytoin are most widely used, when they are available. The problem remains basic logistical support of drug ordering, transport to locales, stock rotation and re-ordering and prevention of pilferage. When these problems are overcome most developing countries will then be in a position to effectively determine whether other antiepileptic drugs and their varying formulations should become available.

SUMMARY: EPILEPSY AS A NATIONAL AND INTERNATIONAL MEDICAL PRIORITY

A recent shift has occured in international health-care priorities. Moving away from acute infectious disease as a main emphasis, international groups such as the WHO and the World Bank now wish to focus on the needs that arise from chronic diseases and 'diseases of affluence', resulting from the adoption of Western habits such as smoking, high fat and protein diets, automobile use etc. Notably, epilepsy is not a priority for these international assistance groups, and few national governments emphasize epilepsy as a health-care priority. The management of paediatric epilepsy in developing countries is immensely complicated by the social and economic realities faced by these nations. Despite these problems, progress is being made in model programmes that choose to adapt, rather than to adopt, Western-style methods of clinical care and research.

The lack of data required to determine a cost–benefit analysis for the prevention and care of seizure patients hampers decision-makers in national health ministries. Given these realities, it is essential that more emphasis be placed on: (1) gathering culturally specific data on the costs and benefits of caring for epilepsy in developing countries; (2) gathering population-based data regarding the incidence, prevalence and prevention of epilepsy; (3) improving widescale education of community health workers and others who can screen for epilepsy and begin first-line medical therapy and patient education; (4) convincing national and regional governments of the need to assure a continuous supply of quality antiepileptic drugs at a local level; (5) making concerted attempts to break cycles of educational, employment and other social discrimination against young epileptics in developing countries, (6) renewing efforts to convince international organizations such as the WHO and the World Bank that epilepsy should be regarded as a higher health priority in long-range health planning; and (7) creating active preventive efforts to reduce important risk factors for epilepsy, in particular head trauma and intracranial infection.

In a world facing seemingly insurmountable economic constraints, political turmoil in many quarters and new health challenges (in particular AIDS), progress in paediatric epilepsy care may need to be measured one child at a time.

REFERENCES

Ajmone-Marsan C & Zivin L (1970) Factors related to the occurrence of typical paroxysmal abnormalities in the EEG records of epileptic patients. *Epilepsia* 11: 361–381.

Alarcon G & Olivares L (1975) Cysticercosis cerebrale. Manifestaciones en un medio de alta prevelencia. *Revista de Investigacion Clinica* 27: 209–215.

Albuquerque M, Alonso NB, Vincenzo NS et al (1991) Multidisciplinary treatment of intractable partial epilepsy. 19th International Epilepsy Congress. *Epilepsia* 32 (supplement 1): 32.

Al Rajeh S, Abomelha A & Awada A (1990) Epilepsy and other convulsive disorders in Saudi Arabia: a prospective study of 1000 consecutive cases. *Acta Neurologica Scandinavica* 82: 341–345.

Annegers JF, Hauser WA, Anderson VE & Kurland LT (1982) The risk of seizure disorder among relatives of patients with childhood onset epilepsy. *Neurology* **32:** 174–179.

Arruda WO (1991) Etiology of epilepsy. A prospective study of 210 cases. *Arquivos de Neuropsiquiatria* **49:** 251–254.

Arseni C & Marinescu V (1974) Epilepsy in cerebral hydatidosis. *Epilepsia* **15:** 45–54.

Avondet M, Castelli Y & Scaremelli A (1991) Psychologic and social adjustment in adolescents with epilepsy. 19th International Epilepsy Congress. *Epilepsia* **32 (supplement 1):** 43.

Aziz H (1989) *Epilepsy and treatment in two community based studies in Pakistan and Turkey.* 18th International Epilepsy Congress, New Delhi, India.

Aziz H, Ali SM & Hasan KZ (1991a) Consanguinity and epilepsy. 19th International Epilepsy Congress. *Epilepsia* **32 (supplement 1):** 64.

Aziz H, Hasan M & Hasan KZ (1991b) Prevalence of epilepsy in children (a population survey report). *Journal of the Pakistan Medical Association* **41:** 134–136.

Bahemuka M & Murungi JH (1989) Tuberculosis of the nervous system. A clinical, radiological and pathological study of 39 consecutive cases in Riyadh, Saudia Arabia. *Journal of the Neurological Sciences* **90:** 67–76.

Bartolomei F, Pellegrino P, Dhiver C et al (1991) Epilepsy seizures in HIV infection. 52 cases. *Presse Medicale* **20:** 2135–2139.

Broadhurst LE, Erickson RL & Kelley PW (1993) Decreases in invasive *Haemophilus influenzae* disease in US Army children, 1984 through 1991. *Journal of the American Medical Association* **268:** 227–231.

Browne TR & Penry JK (1973) Benzodiazepines in the treatment of epilepsy: a review. *Epilepsia* **14:** 277.

Chandy MJ, Rajshekhar V, Ghosh S et al (1991) Single small enhancing CT lesions in Indian patients with epilepsy: clinical, radiological and pathological considerations. *Journal of Neurology, Neurosurgery and Psychiatry* **54:** 702–705.

Chang HT, Wang CW, Yu CF et al (1957) Paragonimiasis. A clinical study of 200 adult cases. *Chinese Medical Journal* **77:** 3–9.

Dada TO (1970) Parasites and epilepsy in Nigeria. *Tropical and Geographical Medicine* **22:** 313–322.

Dancy RD, May M & Cowie RL (1992) Seizures and neurocysticercosis in black men. *South African Medical Journal* **81:** 424–425.

Davis A (1983) A epidemiologia da teniase e da cisticercose. *Journal of Brazilian Medicine* **45:** 9–14.

Dumas M, Grunitzky E, Deiau M et al (1989) Epidemiological study of neurocysticercosis in northern Togo (West Africa). *Acta Leiden* **57:** 191–196.

Editorial (1988) Sodium valproate. *Lancet* **ii:** 1229–1231.

Elechi CA (1991) Default and non-compliance among adult epileptics in Zaria, Nigeria. *Tropical and Geographical Medicine* **33:** 242–245.

Elliot DL, Tolle SW, Goldberg L & Miller JB (1985) Pet-associated illnesses. *New England Journal of Medicine* **313:** 985–995.

Ellison RE, Guvener A, Feksi G et al (1988) A study of approaches to antiepileptic drug treatment in four countries in the developing world. In Dreifuss F et al (eds) *Advances in Epileptology. 17th Epilepsy International Symposium.* New York: Raven Press.

Fan KJ & Pezeshkpour GH (1986) Cerebral sparganosis. *Neurology* **36:** 1249–1251.

Feksi AT & Gatiti SN (1991) Factors determining outcome of epilepsy management: a community follow-up study of 302 patients, 1986–1988. International Epilepsy Congress. *Epilepsia* **32 (supplement 1):** 66.

Feksi AT, Kaamugisha J, Sander JWAS et al (1991a) Comprehensive primary health care antiepileptic drug treatment in rural and semirural Kenya. *Lancet* **337:** 406–409.

Feksi AT, Kaamugisha J, Gatiti S et al (1991b) A comprehensive community epilepsy programme: the Nakuru project. *Epilepsy Research* **8:** 252–259.

Felipe GP, Donnadieu R, Velasco F & Rafael F (1991) Knowledge and attitudes toward epilepsy patients in Mexico. 19th International Epilepsy Congress. *Epilepsia* **32 (supplement 1):** 106.

Gadjusek DC (1978) Introduction of *Taenia solium* into West New Guinea with a note on an epidemic of burns from cysticercus epilepsy in the Ekari people of Wissel Lakes area. *Papua New Guinea Medical Journal* **21:** 329–342.

Gastaut H & Osuntokun BO (1976) Proposals on antiepileptic pharmacotherapy for use in developing countries. *Epilepsia* **17**: 355–260.

Gatiti SM & Feksi AT (1991) Role of lay community workers in providing care for patients with epilepsy. 19th International Epilepsy Congress. *Epilepsia* **32 (supplement 1)**: 32.

Goodridge DMG & Shorvon SD (1983) Epileptic seizures in a population of 60 000. 2: Treatment and prognosis. *British Medical Journal* **287**: 645–647.

Goudsmit J, van der Waals FW & Gadjusek DC (1983) Epilepsy in the Gbawain and Wroughbarh Clan of Grand Basa county, Liberia: the endemic occurrence of 'see-ee' in the native population. *Neuroepidemiology* **2**: 35–44.

Gulati P, Jena A, Tripathi RP & Gupta AE (1991) Magnetic resonance imaging in childhood epilepsy. *Indian Pediatrics* **28**: 761–765.

Gururaj G & Satishchandra P (1992) Correlates of hot water epilepsy in rural South India. A descriptive study. *Neuroepidemiology* **11**: 173–179.

Haddad FS, Risk WS & Jabbour JT (1977) Subacute sclerosing panencephalitis in the Middle East: report of 99 cases. *Annals of Neurology* **1**: 211–216.

Haerer AF, Anderson DW & Schoenberg BS (1986) Prevalence and clinical features of biracial United States population. *Epilepsia* **27**: 66–75.

Hauser WA & Kurland LT (1975) The epidemiology of epilepsy in Rochester, Minnesota, 1935 through 1967. *Epilepsia* **16**: 1–16.

Hauser WA, Anderson VE, Loewenson RB & McRoberts SM (1982) Seizure recurrence after a first unprovoked seizure. *New England Journal of Medicine* **307**: 522–528.

International League Against Epilepsy, Commission on Classification and Terminology (1981) Proposed revision of clinical and electroencephalographic classification of epileptic seizures. *Epilepsia* **22**: 480–501.

International League Against Epilepsy, Commission on Classification and Terminology (1989) Proposal for revised classification of epilepsies and epileptic syndromes. *Epilepsia* **30**: 389–399.

Ismael S (1990) The efficacy of phenobarbital in controlling epilepsy in children. *Paediatrica Indonesiana* **30**: 97–110.

Jain S & Maheshwari MC (1991) A prolonged prospective follow-up study of 306 epileptic patients in New Delhi. *Acta Neurologica Scandinavica* **84**: 471–474.

Janz D & Beck-Mannagetta G (1982) Epilepsy and neonatal seizures in the offspring of parents with epilepsy. In Anderson VE et al (eds) *Genetic basis of epilepsies*, pp 135–143. New York: Raven Press.

Jilek WG & Jilek-Aall LM (1977) The problem of epilepsy in a rural Tanzanian tribe. *African Journal of Medical Sciences* **1**: 305–307.

Kaamugisha J & Feksi AT (1988) Determining the prevalence of epilepsy in the semi-urban population of Nakura, Kenya, comparing two independent methods not apparently used before in epilepsy studies. *Neuroepidemiology* **7**: 115–121.

Kies BM, Handley I, Henochsberg P & Clarke J (1991) Combined medical and psychosocial evaluation of, and assistance to workers with epilepsy. 19th International Epilepsy Congress. *Epilepsia* **32 (supplement 1)**: 30.

Li S, Schoenberg BS, Wang CC et al (1985) Epidemiology of epilepsy in urban areas of the People's Republic of China. *Epilepsia* **26**: 391–394.

McFadyen ML, Miller R, Juta M & Hodgson V (1990) The prevalence of a First-World therapeutic drug monitoring service to the treatment of epilepsy in Third-World conditions. *South African Medical Journal* **78**: 587–590.

Mani KS (1987) *Collaborative epidemiological study on epilepsy in India. Final report of the Bangalore Centre*. Bangalore: National Institute of Mental Health and Neurological Sciences, Bangalore, India.

Mani KS, Mani AJ & Ramesh CK (1975) Hot water epilepsy: a peculiar type of reflex epilepsy. Clinical and electroencephalographic features in 108 cases. *Transactions of the American Neurologists Association* **99**: 224.

Mattson RH, Cramer JA & Collins JF (1985) Comparison of carbamazepine, phenobarbital, phenytoin and primidone in partial and secondary generalized tonic–clonic seizures. *New England Journal of Medicine* **313**: 145–151.

Mausner JS & Kramer S (1985) Population dynamics and health. In Mausner JS & Kramer S (eds) *Epidemiology, An Introductory Text*, pp 239–262. Philadelphia: WB Saunders.

Meinardi H (1988) Epilepsy in developing countries. Part III. In Richens AL, Laidlaw J & Oxley J (eds) *A Textbook of Epilepsy*, pp 528–532. Edinburgh: Churchill Livingstone.

Metrakos JD & Metrakos K (1966) Childhood epilepsy of subcortical (centrencephalic) origin. *Clinical Pediatrics* **5**: 536–542.

Naito H, Wachi M & Nishida M (1987) Clinical effects and plasma concentrations of long-term clonazepam monotherapy in previously untreated epileptics. *Acta Neurologica Scandinavica* **76**: 58–63.

Ogunniyi A & Osuntokun BO (1991) Effectiveness of anticonvulsant therapy in epilepsies in Nigerian Africans. *East African Medical Journal* **68**: 707–713.

Osuntokun BO (1978) Epilepsy in Africa. *Tropical and Geographical Medicine* **30**: 23–32.

Osuntokun BO, Adeuja AOG & Nottidge VA (1987a) Prevalence of epilepsies in Nigerian Africans: a community-based study. *Epilepsia* **28**: 272–279.

Osuntokun BO, Adeuja AO, Schoenberg BS et al (1987b) Neurological disorders in Nigerian Africans: a community-based study. *Acta Neurologica Scandinavica* **75**: 13–21.

Parks-Trusz S & Troxell J (1991) The transition from school to work for young adults with epilepsy. 19th International Epilepsy Congress. *Epilepsia* **32 (supplement 1)**: 30.

Peiris H & Senanayake N (1991) Seizure-related injuries in epileptic patients in a developing country in Asia. 19th International Epilepsy Congress. *Epilepsia* **32 (supplement 1)**: 66.

Placencia M, Suarez J, Crespo F et al (1992) A large-scale study of epilepsy in Ecuador: methodological aspects. *Neuroepidemiology* **11**: 74–84.

Pomata HB, Picco H, Medina C & Waisburg C (1991) Preliminary results in surgical management of intractable epilepsy. *Epilepsia* **32**: 53.

Rogazzo PC, Cendes F, Da Costa et al (1991) Callosotomy in mentally retarded patients with intractable epilepsy: results in different seizure types. *Epilepsia* **32**: 53.

Schier E, Yecunnoamlack T, Tegegne T & Gedlu E (1991) The problem of epilepsy in children and adolescents in developing countries. 19th International Epilepsy Congress. *Epilepsia* **32 (supplement 1)**: 29.

Schoenberg BS (1987) Recent studies of the epidemiology of epilepsy in developing countries: a coordinated program for prevention and control. *Epilepsia* **28**: 721–722.

Scrimgeour EM & Gadjusek DC (1985) Involvement of the central nervous system in *Schistosoma mansoni* and *S. hematobium* infection. *Brain* **108**: 1023–1038.

Shorvon SD & Farmer PJ (1988) Epilepsy in developing countries: a review of epidemiological, sociocultural and treatment aspects. *Epilepsia* **29 (supplement 1)**: S36–S54.

Shorvon SD, Hart YM, Sander JWAS & van Andel F (1991) *The Management of Epilepsy in Developing Countries: and 'ICBERG' manual. International Congress and Symposium*, no. 175, pp 25–28. London: Royal Society of Medicine Services.

Srindharan R, Radhakrishnan K, Asok PP & Mousa ME (1986) Epidemiological and clinical study of epilepsy in Benghazi, Libya. *Epilepsia* **27**: 60–65.

Thomas L (1993) *The Fragile Species*, p 84. New York: Charles Scribner's Sons.

Thompson P & Upton D (1991) Living with intractable epilepsy: impact on family members. 19th International Epilepsy Congress. *Epilepsia* **32 (supplement 1)**: 42.

Tsuboi T & Endo S (1977) Incidence of seizures and EEG abnormalities among offspring of epileptic parents. *Human Genetics* **36**: 173–189.

World Health Organization (1988) *Third Report of the WHO Expert Committee. The Use of Essential Drugs*. Geneva: WHO.

Yang PJ, Berger MD, Cohen ME & Duffner PK (1979) Computer tomography and childhood seizure disorders. *Neurology* **29**: 1084–1088.

Young AC, Borg-Constanze J, Mohr PD & Forbes W (1982) Is routine computerized axial tomographic scanning in epilepsy worthwhile? *Lancet* **ii**: 1446–1447.

5

Non-pharmacological approaches to children's epilepsy

RUBY H. SCHWARTZ

For all children with epilepsy, drugs are but one aspect of management and attention to life-style is all important. Circumstances that need special consideration include:

1. Children who take conventional drugs to control the seizures but need additional measures to minimize the number of seizures.
2. Those who do not respond to conventional pharmacological treatment, either used singularly or in combination in optimal doses.
3. Those children whose parents or guardians totally or partially reject the use of conventional anti-epileptic drugs because of actual or feared side-effects.
4. Children who refuse to take their medication.
5. Children of parents who are reluctant or will not give conventional treatments and turn to complementary medicine including aromatherapy, faith healing, cranial osteopathy, homoeopathy, herbalism, colour therapy and acupuncture.

In this chapter alternative non-pharmacological treatments are discussed (Table 1). Some of these form part of conventional fully accepted medical

Table 1. Non-pharmacological approaches to the treatment of epilepsy.

Diet
    Ketogenic
    Oligoantigenic

Surgery
    Removal of mass of epileptogenic tissue
    Removal of structurally abnormal tissue
    Disconnection procedures

Behavioural therapy

Complementary
    Acupuncture
    Aromatherapy
    Homoeopathy

Baillière's Clinical Paediatrics—
Vol. 2, No. 3, August 1994
ISBN 0–7020–1862–7

practice such as surgery. Western paediatricians have mixed views concerning treatments such as ketogenic diets and, to a greater extent, oligoantigenic diets and behavioural therapy, but are usually prepared to give them a trial in carefully selected cases where conventional drugs have not been fully successful. A proportion of the epilepsies of childhood fail to respond to conventional therapy and it is important that medical practitioners know what other treatments are tried by some parents. When one hears of non-approved therapies that seem to be effective, the obligation on the concerned practitioner is to ensure that they are subject to controlled clinical trials.

Diet

Do children with epilepsy ever need special diets? Occasionally one meets parents who have a quasi-magical attitude to the effect of diet on their offspring's health, resulting in the child being prohibited from eating the food they like or being made to eat something they hate for the sake of seizure control. Special diets in the management or prevention of epilepsy are clearly needed in the management of metabolic disorders including: (1) phenylketonuria and other amino-acidopathies; (2) diabetes mellitus and fits associated with hypoglycaemia; hypoglycaemia is otherwise a problem only in high-risk infants, premature and for small gestational age babies, and those whose mothers have diabetes or other endocrine problems; (3) young children who help themselves to alcoholic drinks as these can cause profound hypoglycaemia. (Hypoglycaemia is otherwise an unusual cause of seizures, although it is always wise to test the blood sugar concentration with a commercial glucose stick test.)

Vitamins and folic acid supplements

The prolonged use of phenytoin, phenobarbitone and primidone have all been associated with folate deficiency (Reynolds, 1967). The same three drugs have also been implicated in the occurrence of metabolic bone disease, particularly when used in high doses and as part of multiple therapy (Dent et al, 1970). It is thus sensible that the diet of all children with epilepsy is reviewed and, if they do not or will not eat vitamin-rich foods, that supplementary vitamins and folic acid be prescribed to maintain an optimal level.

Pyridoxine supplementation is necessary for life in children with pyridoxine-dependent epilepsy, an autosomal recessive disorder (Bankier et al, 1983) associated with seizures at birth or in the first few weeks of life. This condition is rare. The outcome for this condition is generally poor although the earlier treatment is started the better.

Fibre

The proportion of fibre in the diet is controversial. Very high-fibre diets may interfere with the absorption of drugs, especially slow-release tablets, and result in subsequent loss of seizure control (Jeavons and Aspinall, 1985). A more commonly seen phenomenon, for which there is no documented explanation, is the exacerbation of seizures in children suffering from severe constipation, particularly in the 24 h before defaecation.

Aspartame

Aspartame, a commonly used sugar substitute, has been reported in provocation doses to exacerbate EEG spike-wave discharges in children with generalized absence epilepsy. It is not known whether small frequent amounts over long periods cause similar effects and whether children with other types of seizure are similarly affected (Camfield et al, 1992). At present the consensus is not to prohibit aspartame-containing foods in the diet of children with epilepsy.

Provoking factors in childhood epilepsy

The threshold of cerebral excitability may be modified by factors such as hyperventilation, hyperthermia, the ingestion of alcohol, metabolic disorders, including hypocalcaemia and hypoglycaemia, and extreme physical or emotional stress, particularly when accompanied by sleep deprivation. A detailed history may reveal specific provoking factors, and avoidance of these may decrease the risk of seizures.

Fever frequently exacerbates a seizure disorder. Similar precautions should be taken to those recommended to parents of children who have febrile convulsions. Heavy clothing should be removed, patients should be given regular cool fluids when pyrexial and, if necessary, regular antipyretic agents such as paracetamol. Fans blowing air directly on the patient should be avoided as venoconstriction results in ineffective heat loss from the skin and the core temperature may rise; tepid sponging too is no longer recommended for the same reason.

Flicker-induced epilepsy

In this type of epilepsy, seizures are provoked by flickering natural or artificial light. It is the commonest of the true reflex epileptic seizures and accounts for seizures in about 3–5% of people with epilepsy. The condition appears most commonly between the ages of 6 and 15 years; females are more frequently affected (Eeg-Olofsson, 1985). Changes are seen on the EEG during photostimulation. The attacks may occur under natural conditions, for example driving down a tree-lined road in bright sunlight or the play of light on water or snow or reflected from a brilliant object. These attacks may be alleviated by covering one eye or wearing true polarized sunglasses when out of doors on a sunny day. These spectacles have to be specially ordered. Polaroid or other types of tinted spectacles do not help.

Television-induced epilepsy is the commonest type of photosensitive epilepsy (O'Donohoe, 1994). Attacks can be reduced by ensuring that the patient watches the television in a well-lit room, preferably with a small illuminated table-light on top of the set. The patient should be at least 2.5 m away from the set and should avoid approaching the television to adjust it or change channels. Should it be necessary to approach the set, one eye should be covered; an autochanger is advisable. The best televisions for such children are small (35-cm screen) colour sets with a good aerial; poor-copy 'pirated' videos are a real hazard.

Repetitive flickering of lights at discothèques may also provoke seizures in sensitive children. Although avoidance is the best policy, that may be resistible advice. The second best advice is to suggest that the affected person be accompanied by someone who is aware of the diagnosis and capable of ensuring safety should a seizure occur. Covering one eye may prevent a seizure should the lights start to flash unexpectedly.

Recently, concern has been raised about the use of hand-held computer games, such as Nintendo and SEGA. These devices now carry a health and safety warning and should be used with care in children with photosensitivity. The duration of play should be limited to avoid tiredness.

Children with photosensitive epilepsy should be allowed to undertake computer studies at school provided they use a proper visual display unit (VDU) screen which 'refreshes' the picture at least 50 times per second. The latest types of screen refresh at up to 100 times per second and should not cause seizures in photosensitive individuals. Modern VDU screens of the VGA (video graphics array) (or, better, SVGA, super video graphics array) type have a rapid refresh rate; matrix-type screens on modern notebook computers do not seem to cause problems. Photosensitve children should not use standard televisions as computer monitors. Since many jobs now involve some use of VDUs, it is vital that children with epilepsy learn to use computers. Parents should be assured that special schools for children with epilepsy in the UK are liberally equipped with computers.

Other reflex epilepsies

These are extremely rare. Seizures may be triggered by particular mental activity such as hearing or performing music, reading, writing, physical actions such as a light touch on the head, specific visual or auditory imagery, or even the performance of mathematical calculations. Visual imagery may play a role in seizures initiated by computer games. An alternative approach is deconditioning to the particular causal stimulus (Forster et al, 1969).

SPECIFIC DIETS

Ketogenic diets

Ketogenic diets have been used in the treatment of epilepsy since the turn of the century. They were developed following the observation by Guelpa and Marie (1911) that seizures ceased during absolute fasting but recurred once food was reintroduced. Wilder (1921) suggested that the chemical changes found in starvation could be produced for longer periods using a diet high in fat and low in protein and carbohydrates. This subsequently became known as the ketogenic diet.

The original diets recommended by Wilder and Helmholz (1921) and more recently by Livingston (1972) are based on the consumption of a high proportion of long-chain saturated fats. Many children, however, find such a diet restrictive and unpalatable, and compliance is poor. With the advent of more effective antiepileptic drugs, dietary treatments ceased to be popular, but over recent years it has been recognized that they are worth trying in those children who do not respond adequately to conventional antiepileptic drugs and may appeal to those parents who are reluctant to give drugs. Huttenlocher (1976) introduced a new diet based on medium-chain triglyceride (MCT) oil, which had also been shown to induce ketosis and produce similar changes to the original diets. This diet was said to be cheaper, less restrictive, and more palatable than the original diet. The clinical and metabolic effects of three different ketogenic diets were studied by Schwartz et al (1989a,b): (1) the original ketogenic diet; (2) the MCT diet; and (3) a combination of both (modified MCT diet). The diets are summarized in Table 2.

Table 2. Ketogenic diets.

	MCT diet	Modified MCT	Classical
Calculation of daily food requirements	RDI	RDI	75 kcal/kg body-weight 1 g protein/kg body-weight
MCT oil	60%	30%	36 k calories from long chain saturated fats to 4 k calories from protein & carbohydrates
Long-chain saturated fats	11% (naturally occurring in foods)	41%	
Protein	10%	10%	
Carbohydrate	19%	19%	
Vitamins	Ketovite (supplements)	Ketovite (supplements)	Ketovite (supplements)

MCT, Medium-chain triglycerides; RDI, recommended daily intake.

Original ketogenic diet

The fat source is from naturally occurring saturated and unsaturated fatty acids. The number of calories and their distribution may be ascertained from precalculated data provided by Livingston (1972) or Mike (1965) (Table 2). Alternatively, they may be calculated individually using the following data:

1. Recommended total number of kcal/day = weight of patient in kilograms × the number of kilocalories needed to meet growth requirements-weight (in our calculations we have used 75 kcal per kg per day.)
2. 4 g fat contributes 36 kcal
3. 1 g of either carbohydrate or protein contributes 4 kcal

4. 1 dietary unit consisting of 4 g fat and 1 g protein and carbohydrate therefore contributes 40 kcal
5. The daily protein requirement to maintain adequate growth is 1 g per kg per day

From these facts the composition of the diet is worked out as follows:

1. Total kcal/day = weight × 75 kcal/kg
2. Total number of dietary units = total no. kcal divided by 40.
3. Amount of fat = number of dietary units × 4
4. Amount of protein + carbohydrate = number of dietary units × 1
5. Amount of protein = 1 g per kg
6. Amount of carbohydrate = amount of protein + carbohydrate less the amount of protein

With this diet the daily calorific total is divided between three equal meals, breakfast, lunch and supper, each of which conforms to the strict 4:1 ratio.

To help parents, a system of basic meal exchanges has been devised for each child according to the daily allowance; this provides a useful means of constructing a diet that includes the child's specific likes and dislikes. In this way, satisfactory toddler, children's and adult meat or vegetarian diets can be devised. Parents are asked to attempt to ensure that the complete meal is eaten and that no food is carried over to subsequent meals, so that the strict 4:1 ratio can be maintained throughout.

The medium-chain triglyceride diet

The major fat source is MCT oil, a fractionated coconut oil containing predominantly C8 and C10 saturated fatty acids incorporated into the diet as an emulsion in skimmed milk and also used as oil. It is currently available on prescription in the UK as both an oil and an emulsion (Liquigen), which is much simpler to use.

With this diet the total daily calories are based on the recommended daily intake, obtained from dietetic tables calculated according to the child's age. The calories are distributed between fat, protein and carbohydrate, as shown in Table 2.

This diet has the advantage that the total intake can be distributed throughout the day. Since it contains more carbohydrates, children tend to prefer it. Carbohydrate taken on its own without fat, as with snacks between meals, has an antiketogenic effect and the clinical benefits may be reversed. Sweets and chocolates should be avoided completely, but potato chips and crisps are permissible as they contain both fat and carbohydrates.

The abrupt introduction of 60% of the calories as MCT oil results in nausea, vomiting and abdominal discomfort. For this reason the amount of oil should be increased gradually over several days until the full amount is incorporated or maximum tolerance is reached.

The modified MCT diet

The modified MCT diet has also been used in some patients who have found the MCT diet unacceptable. The modified diet contains less oil and is based on an exchange system for proteins and carbohydrate and a fixed amount of fat each day. The proportion of each type of food is shown in Table 2. The amounts of oil and long-chain saturated and unsaturated fats can be modified according to individual taste and tolerance.

With all diets, 'free foods'—particularly vegetables and fruit—can be taken freely. These are useful in increasing bulk and adding flavour. Details should be discussed with dieticians experienced in the establishment and supervision of these diets. They need great skill as most children have very distinct food fads and special likes and dislikes. An experienced dietician will be expert in devising treats such as water ices from diabetic fruit drinks and modified ice cream. In the long run, however, only the motivated family and placid child stick to the diet; there is no point in harassing those who cannot keep it going.

Vitamin supplements

Although the ketogenic diet is rich in fat-soluble vitamins A and D, it is deficient in the water-soluble vitamins of the B and C complexes. All children receiving a ketogenic diet should be started on vitamin supplements in the form of a full multivitamin preparation such as Ketovite tablets (one tablet three times daily) and Ketovite liquid (5 ml daily) or other equivalents. The diet is relatively deficient in minerals, so younger children in particular should be started on mineral supplements. Additional calcium is not given routinely to older children provided they were previously taking a balanced diet and serum calcium levels are monitored.

Schwartz et al (1989a,b) studied 55 children with many different types of epilepsy who had failed to respond to conventional treatments in full dosage. The majority had drop attacks, including head nods, bilateral massive epileptiform myoclonus and atonic attacks. All three types of diet were tried and all were associated with a reduction of seizure frequency (Table 3). No child regressed while taking the diet. There was no significant association between the seizure type and the success of dietary treatment.

The high fat diet was palatable to all children but its preparation was found to be the most complicated and expensive. Large quantities of MCT oil were unpalatable to all age groups, particularly older children and adults, and many of those who initially accepted the oil subsequently rejected it.

The short-term safety of the diets has been established. Very few complications are encountered. Nausea, vomiting and abdominal distension occurs in approximately half the patients while the MCT diet is being established.

Table 3. Clinical response to ketogenic diets.

Diet	Reduction in seizure frequency		Total no. of studies
	>50%	<50%	
Original 4:1	22	2	24
MCT	21	6	27
Modified MCT	8	4	12

This can be overcome by temporarily reducing the amount of oil and then increasing it again more gradually. Steatorrhoea may occur while on the classical ketogenic diet, but this resolves when the total fat content of the diet is reduced. Drowsiness occurs in about 25% of children while being established on any of the three diets, but this resolved spontaneously after a few days and did not cause major problems.

Urinary ketones should be monitored regularly with Ketostix. Levels tend to be lower in the morning and higher in the evening. Fluctuations in the concentrations of urinary ketones are to be expected while children are receiving the diet; this does not appear to reflect seizure control. Frequently ketone levels fall in the prodomal phase of an intercurrent illness, and this may be clinically relevant. Growth is not affected as long as the protein and overall calorie requirements of the child are supplied. Livingstone (1972) felt that there was no increased risk of coronary artery disease and atheroma as long as the overall calorie requirement was followed, but there is no long-term evidence to confirm this. Visual disturbances and renal calculi have been reported. The latter are thought to be due to poor fluid intake (Hopkins and Lynch, 1970; Hertzberg et al, 1990). Before starting the diet it must be established that the child is not milk intolerant. Chronic gastrointestinal problems are not a contraindication (Rosental et al, 1990).

There has been one documented case of a child developing severe mucocutaneous and subcutaneous infection with *Staphylococcus aureus*. Subsequent investigation has shown that there may be impaired neutrophil function in children with seizures treated with the ketogenic diet (Woody et al, 1989).

Although much of the research on ketogenic diets has been based on the use of saturated fats or medium-chain glycerides, corn oil can be used as a substitute for MCT oil. Corn oil is much less expensive and more readily available than MCT oil. It is also better tolerated and appears to be free from clinical toxicity. It can be substituted for MCT oil in the calculation in either an MCT or a modified MCT diet (Woody et al, 1988).

Possible mode of action

Despite extensive studies, the mechanism by which the ketogenic diet acts remains unknown. It is possible that two mechanisms exist. Ketone bodies may act as antiepileptic factors in their own right and thus explain why some children's seizure control varies with fluctuations in ketone levels. Alternatively the effect may be mediated by changes in nerve cell lipid membrane, resulting in decreased neurological excitation or in the local production or clearance of neurotransmitters.

Oligoantigenic diet

Interest in food allergy as a cause or a contributor to the severity of epilepsy was rekindled following the reports by Egger and co-workers (1983, 1985, 1989) that children with migraine and hyperactive behaviour who also had seizures showed an improvement during dietary therapy. Improvement was noted particularly if the children had associated migraine, hyperkinetic behaviour or both.

To establish which foods were involved 46 children aged from 2 to 16 years were established on an oligoantigenic diet (Table 4) for 2 weeks (Egger et al, 1989). Those who did not improve were offered a second oligoantigenic diet which consisted of food not included in the first diet. If the patient responded, foods were reintroduced singly at the rate of one per week. Those foods tolerated without symptoms were maintained in the diet. If there was any recurrence in symptoms, this food was eliminated. Nutritional adequacy and patient preference were considered in all cases. EEG studies were carried out on children with several different types of epilepsy and varying seizure frequency before and after receiving the diet, using a double-

Table 4. Foods permitted in the oligoantigenic diet.

Meat	(lamb and chicken)
Carbohydrates	(potato and rice)
Fruit	(banana and apple)
Vegetables	(cabbage, sprouts, cauliflower, broccoli, cucumber, celery, carrots and parsnips)
Water	
Salt, pepper	
Calcium	
Vitamins	
Pure herbs	

blind procedure. No child with epilepsy alone without associated symptoms such as headaches, abdominal pain or hyperkinetic behaviour improved with the diet, whereas a marked improvement was seen in those with more than one problem, both in seizure control and in the frequency of associated symptoms. Forty-two foods provoked symptoms, of which 21 provoked seizures. Cow's milk was the most common provoking substance, although tartrazine, benzoic acid and chocolate were postulated as causes. Other common provoking foods included citrus fruits and wheat. The median reaction time for the recurrence of symptoms was 2 days (Egger et al, 1989).

Wurtman (1983) suggested that the neurotransmitters involved might be derived from the gut and that intracerebral levels of amino acid-derived neurotransmitters can be affected by dietary precursors. Opiate-like peptides have been discovered in milk and wheat (Brantl and Teschenmacher, 1979; Klee et al, 1979) and implicated in the pathophysiology of epileptic seizures (Frenk et al, 1979).

Oligoantigenic diets need close supervision. They should be undertaken only in children who have both migraine and epilepsy, particularly if the child is drug resistant. They are socially disruptive and expensive. Dietary monitoring is essential to exclude malnutrition (Tripp et al, 1979) and care needs to be taken to avoid anaphylaxis or status epilepticus on the reintroduction of foods (David, 1984).

HOLISTIC APPROACH

Behavioural therapies

Lay opinion often associates stress with seizures, but how true is this? EEG studies show that neurophysiological changes can be stress induced. Children are sometimes able to control the frequency of attacks to some degree. Evidence of this should always be sought when questioning children about seizures. Some children are able to induce seizures, particularly those who are exceptionally light sensitive, have frequent seizures and a personality disorder often associated with low intelligence. The most common method is by rapidly moving a hand in front of the face while looking at the sun or another bright light. Most cannot give an explanation for their behaviour, although pleasure and escape from stress or boredom may be factors. This type of epilepsy is difficult to treat and it is often necessary to help the family rather than the child (Betts, 1982).

Some patients with sensory or motor epilepsy can inhibit their attacks once they have started, either by vigorous sensory stimulation of the involved area or by brisk muscular activity. Physical exercise has been shown to raise the seizure threshold and may reduce the likelihood of seizures occurring.

Video-telemetry used with EEG may give valuable advice about the role of stress and seizures. Stressful events may increase the amount of abnormal activity, as do boredom and inactivity in children. Fatigue, sleep deprivation, overtaxing intellectual effort and hyperventilation are important precipitants, whereas physical exercise and interesting intellectual work reduces the number of seizures. Psychological methods may be helpful in treatment by reducing anxiety (Mattison et al, 1970).

Psychological treatments have been reviewed by Mostofsky and Balaschat (1977). They include operant conditioning (reward of non-seizure behaviour and punishment of seizure behaviour) desensitization, relaxation, psychotherapy, habituation and biofeedback.

Biofeedback is a method of helping patients to change certain physiological functions of which they are normally unaware. Electronic devices are used to pick up signals from parts of the body, e.g. muscle, blood pressure, heart rate or brain. These signals are converted to visual or auditory signals which the patient can recognize and learn to alter. Its clinical uses have been described by Basmajian (1979). Research was initially undertaken on cows who were taught to enhance the amount of sensorimotor rhythm in their EEG; they became seizure resistant when exposed to noxious chemicals (Sterman, 1973; Sterman & MacDonald, 1978). Other workers have been less successful with this technique and the role of biofeedback in the management of children with epilepsy remains unclear.

Holistic approaches are being studied extensively in many units, and methods are being sought to break the vicious circle of fear of the next seizure and subsequent reinforcement. Methods used by Betts (among others) include sensory stimuli, relaxation techniques, imagery and cognitive techniques. By learning how to recognize and assess specific learning factors involved in the triggering and inhibition of the epileptic seizure, individual treatment strategies can be devised. This approach can be applied to child patients and have been used by Dahl and colleagues (1988) in Sweden. '*Taking Control of Your Epilepsy: A Workbook for Patients and Professionals*' published in 1987 resulted from clinical research by the Andres–Reiter Epilepsy Program and is aimed at increasing control of seizures and improving the quality of life through biofeedback training and self-discovery. These approaches were discussed at the Epilepsy Europe Conference in 1992 in Glasgow and show how methods other than the pharmacological treatment of epilepsy are becoming important in patient management (Creggans et al, 1992).

COMPLEMENTARY MEDICINE

Some patients of children with epilepsy are reluctant to use any therapeutic methods, particularly the conventional antiepileptic drugs routinely accepted in orthodox medicine, and turn to alternative therapies. Herbalism is one of the oldest of these treatments. Two herbs in particular have long been used by herbalists in the management of epilepsy. Hyssop (*Hyssopus officinalis*) is said to be helpful in the management of anxiety states, hysteria and petit mal epilepsy. It is taken either as an infusion or a tincture. Skull cap (*Scutellaria laterifolia*) has a reputation as a relaxant of nervous tension and is also said to have a renewing and reviving effect on the CNS. This herb has been used in the treatment of seizures, hysterical states and epilepsy as an infusion or tincture (Hoffman, 1988).

[*It cannot be stressed too strongly that these herbs should not be used in the treatment of epilepsy—editor.*]

Another ancient form of treatment for epilepsy is based on traditional Chinese medicine. The Chinese view the universe as an infinite network of interweaving energy flows which, in disease, become disjointed. Several factors influence the occurrence and remission of disease: external factors, such as climate and acupuncture; internal factors such as emotions; and factors that are neither internal nor external and are influenced by life-style. In the treatment of epilepsy the aim of treatment is to clear the orifices of the head. The methods used during the course of the seizure and those used between seizures are different. Different points on the body have been related to different sorts of seizures and whether they occur during the day or night; the treatment depends on the type of seizure experienced by the patient (Ross, 1985).

Homoeopathy may be practised on its own or in conjunction with conventional medication. Individual therapists use different drugs and these may include: Hyoscyanus in various strengths, Bufo 30, Belladonna 30, Cuprum metallicum, and Stramonium. The practice of homoeopathy dates from nineteenth century Germany and is based on the premise that the symptoms of a disease are evidence of a process going on in the body in response to a disease. The homoeopathic practitioner attempts to promote the further development of the symptoms in order to accelerate the body's natural healing properties. Minute doses of a substance that, if given in excess, would produce symptoms of the disorder—in the case of epilepsy provoke seizures—form the basis of therapy.

Aromatherapy is thought to act by reducing stress and anxiety and it is said to be beneficial in some patients.

The author advises great caution regarding the use of herbal medicine, acupuncture, homoeopathy and aromatherapy in the treatment of epilepsy. None of these methods has been subject to conventional trials of efficacy; their use may distance a patient from a practitioner of orthodox medicine and well-proven treatments may be ignored. Herbal medicines, in particular, may be completely unstandardized in composition and potentially harmful.

A conventionally trained doctor may be greatly taxed by a parent who refuses drug therapy. Many parents with handicapped children make a round of unorthodox practitioners, often paying large sums of money in the process. Doctors should not hesitate to ask whether other types of practitioner are involved in the care of their child; sometimes parents withdraw or change medication or add other unconventional substances that may have a cumulative effect. Circumstances can arise when withdrawal of conventional medication is tantamount to child abuse. Here the doctor must seek appropriate advice according to National Child Protection Guidelines, yet not withdrawing their responsibility for the child's well-being.

SURGERY

Sir Victor Horsley is credited with the introduction of modern surgical procedures for the treatment of epilepsy in the late nineteenth century. Stereotactic surgery began during the 1930s and 1940s. The temporal lobe was identified as the most frequent location for partial seizures and temporal lobectomy produced minimal neurological impairment in most patients. Anterior temporal lobectomy gradually became an accepted treatment for serious drug-resistant epilepsy. Initially it was used predominantly in adults, but recently there has been a greater tendency to operate on children with intractable seizures. The advent of new investigative procedures has made detailed preoperative assessment both essential and accurate.

Surgery can help to control seizures in two ways. The first is to treat focal brain pathology, although difficulties may be encountered in locating the specific focus or there may not appear to be a direct link between the pathology and the focus. The second is to influence brain function to prevent or restrict the propagation of the discharge (Polkey, 1989).

Surgical treatment should be considered for children who have severe disabling seizures refractory to antiepileptic drugs, defined as uncontrolled over a 2–4-year period of treatment with appropriate anticonvulsant drugs in optimum doses. Many of these patients have partial seizures. The child should not have a progressive neurological disease and the prognosis for spontaneous recovery should be poor. The aims of surgery are to remove pathology when there is a primary focus, to disconnect a focus from the rest of the brain where the removal of the primary focus is not possible, and to reduce the mass of neurones that behave abnormally. Problems potentially amenable to surgery include:

1. Pathology such as tumour or arterio-venous malformation
2. Congenital disorder—Aicardi syndrome, Rasmussen syndrome etc.
3. Landau–Kleffner syndrome

Three main types of surgery are used: focal corticectomy, hemispherectomy and corpus callosotomy.

The indications for each type of operation are shown in Table 5. The optimum age for performing surgery is unknown. Some feel that surgery for epilepsy should be carried out at an early age to prevent the psychological and neurological damage that may occur following long-term seizures (Silfvenius et al, 1989). Others deprecate an aggressive approach and teach that spontaneous remission may yet occur, thus avoiding surgery (Ashkenasi and Carter-Snead, 1989).

Investigation

Before admitting a child for surgery, detailed presurgical evaluation is necessary (Table 6). A detailed history is required in an attempt to elicit any

Table 5. Surgical treatment.

Operation	Indication
Focal cortical resection	
Temporal	Partial seizures
Extratemporal	Localized seizure focus clinically and electrographically/ radiologically
Corpus callosotomy	Intractable, generalized tonic–clonic, atonic or myoclonic seizures
Hemispherectomy	Arising from widespread areas in one damaged hemisphere; Rasmussen syndrome

Table 6. Assessment for surgery.

General
History (including drug history)
Medical and neurological assessment (including visual field assessment)
Psychiatric evaluation
Social assessment

Investigations
EEG and telemetry
Computed tomography with and without contrast
Magnetic resonance imaging
Positron emission tomography
Cerebral angiography
Left and right cerebral amytal testing
Subdural grid placement
Intraoperative functional mapping with epidural, subdural and depth electrodes

incidents that may give rise to epilepsy, as well as a full drug history. The level of social and intellectual functioning should be assessed. The history should also include a clear account of the seizure pattern, both from the patient and an independent observer. An extensive neurological examination follows, together with psychiatric and psychological assessments.

This is followed by neuroradiological magnetic resonance imaging, to produce information about brain structure and pathology including arteriovenous malformations, hamartomas and slow-growing glial tumours. Positron emission tomography, which displays functional abnormalities by measuring regional cerebral blood flow and regional cerebral metabolic rate, may sometimes demonstrate focal lesions potentially amenable to surgery (Chugani et al, 1990) but undetectable by other neuroradiological measures.

Base-line EEGs, together with continuous EEG video-telemetry evoked responses and visual field testing, are also important. If the patient is considered appropriate for surgery, cerebral angiography is performed: amylobarbital is injected into the posterior cerebral artery to determine cerebral dominance for speech and memory, as language may be affected following temporal lobectomy (Jack et al, 1988). In children undergoing focal cortical resection further functional details are obtained with the help of subdural or epidural electrodes (Larkins and Hahn, 1989). These may also be of help in locating speech centres and determining motor and sensory function. Depth electrodes—thin wires with multiple contacts for recording EEGs—are implanted stereotactically into cerebral structures, and subdural electrodes are placed over the surface of the brain.

Types of surgery

Resective operations on the temporal lobe are used most frequently. Very selective procedures, such as selective amygdalo-hippocampectomy described by Wieser (1986), result in maximum seizure control with the minimum risk of cerebral damage. Extratemporal resections may also be undertaken.

Major resections involve the removal of several lobes or most or all of the cerebral hemisphere. They tend to be undertaken in patients with substantial physical handicap often accompanied by considerable intellectual deficit, and should not be undertaken if there is significant risk of increasing the child's physical or intellectual problems.

Functional operations include callosal section which, if restricted to the anterior two thirds, results in minimal complications. Williamson (1985) suggested that this type of surgery is helpful in two groups of patients: those with unilateral hemisphere disease and those with severe generalized epilepsies such as Lennox–Gastaut syndrome.

Results

Criteria used to assess the results of surgery include (Polkey, 1989):

1.   Freedom from, or significant control of, seizures.

2. Complications of surgery, including intellectual and behavioural changes.
3. Mortality in the short and long term.
4. Social and behavioural improvements.

The outcome following focal resection is generally good. The best results are obtained in patients with identifiable lesions and a corresponding seizure focus on EEG, especially with temporal lobe lesions (Cascino et al, 1990; Wyllie, 1991).

The results of temporal lobectomy are said to be better in children than in adults (Henrikson, 1988), with good results reported in between 67 and 85% of children undergoing the procedure (Ashkenasi and Carter-Snead, 1989). The main concern following temporal lobectomy is the effect on language, hence the importance of language mapping before resection. Behavioural problems have also been documented.

The timing of the operation is also significant in order to obtain optimum seizure control with minimal functional and personality problems after operation (Gillingham, 1988).

When major resection was first introduced (Krynauw, 1950) there was very high morbidity and mortality in between one third and one quarter of patients from late complications associated with chronic or delayed bleeding (Falconer and Wilson, 1969). However, in many, particularly patients with infantile hemiplegia and drug resistance seizures, who had behavioural disorders there was an 80% seizure relief with an improvement in behaviour (Wilson, 1970; Rasmussen, 1987). As a result, modified major resectional procedures have been devised, resulting in up to 80% of patients becoming seizure-free with few delayed complications.

A particularly good response has been seen in Rasmussen's encephalitis, a condition characterized by the onset of unilateral focal motor seizures, usually in childhood and occasionally in adolescents, followed by a progressive hemiparesis within 2–4 years. The disease process usually progresses rapidly. In advanced cases there is a good response to hemispherectomy (Rasmussen, 1978). Morrell and co-workers (1989) suggested a further surgical procedure—multiple subpial transection—in which the horizontal cortical connections are divided to reduce propagation of the epileptic discharge, but the vertical fibres by which voluntary movement is initiated are preserved.

The current indications for the use of callosectomy are empirical and complex. Williamson (1985) described a series in which 75% of patients with unilateral hemisphere disease achieved an 80% reduction in seizure frequency, and more than 50% of children with generalized epilepsies showed an 80% reduction in the number of seizures. Partial complex seizures are least affected by the operation. After anterior section there may be periods of mutism, incontinence and limb weakness lasting between a few days and weeks, although these generally resolve. The neuropsychological sequelae of anterior, posterior and complete section have been well documented, but are not necessarily of practical significance (Spencer, 1988).

The surgical treatment of children is complicated and requires very careful, time-consuming and complex evaluations; it can be carried out only in fully equipped special centres. Surgery can dramatically improve the seizure control and quality of life for patients and should be considered when other measures are either unsuitable or are failing.

REFERENCES

Ashkenasi A & Carter-Snead O (1989) Epileptic syndromes and their therapy. *Current Opinion in Pediatrics* **1(2):** 269–277.

Bankier A, Turner M & Hopkins IJ (1983) Pyridoxine dependent seizures—a wider clinical spectrum. *Archives of Disease in Childhood* **58:** 415–418

Basmajian JB (1979) *Biofeedback: Principles and Practice for Clinicians*. Baltimore: Williams & Wilkins.

Betts TA (1982) Psychiatry and epilepsy. In Laidlaw J & Richens A (eds) *A Textbook of Epilepsy*, pp 227–270. Edinburgh: Churchill Livingstone.

Brantl, V & Teschenmacher HA (1979) A material with opioid activity in bovine milk and milk products. *Naunyn-Schmiedebergs Archives of Pharmacology* **306:** 301–304.

Camfield PR, Camfield CS, Dooley JM et al (1992) Aspartame exacerbates electroencephalography spike-wave discharge in children with generalized absence epilepsy: a double-blind controlled study. *Neurology* **42:** 1000–1003.

Cascino GD, Kelly PJ, Hirshorn KA et al (1990) Stereotactic resection of intra-axial cerebral lesions in partial epilepsy. *Mayo Clinic Proceedings* **65:** 1053–1060.

Chugani HT, Shields WD, Shewmon DA et al (1990) Infantile spasms: I PET identifies focal cortical dysgenesis in cryptogenic cases for surgical treatment. *Annals of Neurology* **27:** 406–413.

Creggans S (1992) A review of psychoanalytical literature on epileptic seizures. *Seizure* **1 (supplement A).**

Dahl U, Mehin L & Leissner P (1988) Effects of behavioural intervention on epileptic seizure behaviour and paroxysmal activity: a systemic replication of 3 cases of children with intractable epilepsy. *Epilepsia* **29:** 172–183.

David TJ (1984) Anaphylactic shock during elimination diets in severe atopic eczema. *Archives of Disease in Childhood* **59:** 983–986.

Dent CE, Richens A, Rowe DJF et al (1970) Osteomalacia with long term anticonvulsant therapy in epilepsy. *British Medical Journal* **4:** 69–72.

Eeg-Olofsson O (1985) Types of epilepsy in the young school child: stress flicker and nocturnal seizures. In Ross E & Reynolds E (eds) *Paediatric Perspectives on Epilepsy*, pp 103–110. Chichester: John Wiley.

Egger J, Wilson J, Carter CM et al (1983) Oligo-antigenic diet in epilepsy. *Lancet* **ii:** 865–869.

Egger J, Carter CM, Graham PJ et al (1985) A controlled trial of oligo-antigenic diet treatment in the hyperkinetic syndrome. *Lancet* **i:** 940–945.

Egger J, Carter CM, Soothill JF et al (1989) Oligo-allergenic diet treatment of children with epilepsy and migraine. *Journal of Pediatrics* **114:** 51–58.

Falconer MA & Wilson PJE (1969) Complications related to delayed haemorrhage after hemispherectomy. *Journal of Neurosurgery* **30:** 413–426.

Forster FM, Hanastia P, Cleeland CS et al (1969) A case of voice induced epilepsy treated by conditioning. *Neurology (Minneapolis)* **19:** 325–331.

Frenk H, Engel J Jr, Ackerman RF et al (1979) Endogenous opioids may mediate postictal behavioural depression in amygdaloid kindled rats. *Brain Research* **167:** 435–440.

Gillingham FJ (1988) Surgical treatment of epilepsy, restoration of personality. *Acta Neurochirurgica Supplementum* **44:** 102–105.

Guelpa G & Marie A (1911) La lutte contre l'epilepsie par la desintoxication et par la rééducation alimentaire. *Revue de Therapie Medico-Chirurgicale* **78:** 8–13.

Helmholz HF (1921) The treatment of epilepsy in childhood. Five years' experience with the ketogenic diet. *Journal of the American Medical Association* **88:** 2028–2032.

Henrikson O (1988) Surgical treatment of epilepsy: clinical aspects in children. *Acta Neurologica Scandinavica Supplementum* **117:** 47–51.

Hertzberg GZ, Firush BA, Kinsman SL et al (1990) Urolithiasis associated with ketogenic diets. *Journal of Pediatrics* **117(5)**: 743–745.

Hoffman D (1988) *Holistic Herbal*. Shaftesbury, Dorset: Element Books.

Hopkins IJ & Lynch BC (1970) Use of ketogenic diet in epilepsy in childhood. *Australian Paediatric Journal* **6**: 25–29.

Huttenlocher PR (1976) Ketonemia and seizures: metabolic and anti-convulsant effects of two ketogenic diets in childhood epilepsy. *Pediatric Research* **10**: 536–540.

Jack CR, Nichols DA, Sharbrough FW et al (1988) Selective posterior cerebral artery amytal test for evaluating memory function before surgery for temporal lobe seizure. *Radiology* **168**: 787–793.

Jeavons PM & Aspinall A (1985) *The Epilepsy Reference Book*, p 64. London: Harper and Row.

Klee WA, Zioudrou & Streaty RA (1979) Exorphins: peptides with opioid activity isolated from wheat gluten and their possible role in the aetiology of schizophrenia. In Usdin E, Bunney WE & Kline NS (eds) *Endorphins in Mental Health Research*, pp 209–218. New York: Oxford University Press.

Krynauw RA (19850) Infantile hemiplegia treated by removing a cerebral hemisphere. *Journal of Neurology, Neurosurgery and Psychiatry* **13**: 243–267.

Larkins MV & Hahn JF (1989) Epilepsy surgery in children and young adults the Cleveland clinic experience. *Cleveland Clinic Journal of Medicine* **56 (supplement 2)**: 3266–5288.

Livingston S (1972) Dietary treatment of epilepsy. In *Comprehensive Management of Epilepsy in Infancy, Childhood and Adolescence*, pp 380–405. Springfield, Illinois: CC Thomas.

Mostofsky DI & Balaschat BA (1977) Psychobiological control of seizures. *Psychological Bulletin* **84**: 723–750.

Mattison RH, Heninger GR & Gallagner BB (1970) Seizure and stress: psychophysiological precipitants of seizures in epileptics. *Neurology (Minneapolis)* **20**: 407.

Mike EM (1965) Practical guide and dietary management of children with seizures using the ketogenic diet. *American Journal of Clinical Nutrition* **17**: 399.

Morrell F, Whisler WW & Bleck TP (1989) Multiple subpial transection: a new approach to the surgical treatment of focal epilepsy. *Journal of Neurosurgery* **70**: 231–239.

O'Donohoe NV (1994) Reflex epilepsy. In *Epilepsies of Childhood*, pp 139–145. Oxford: Butterworth–Heinemann.

Polkey CE (1989) Surgical treatment of chronic epilepsy. In Trimble M (ed.) *Chronic Epilepsy, its Prognosis and Management*, pp 189–208. Chichester: J Wiley.

Rasmussen T (1978) Further observations on the syndrome of chronic encephalitis with epilepsy. *Applied Neurophysiology* **41**: 1–12.

Rasmussen T (1987) Cortical resection for multilobe epileptogenic lesions. In Weser HG & Elger C (eds) *Presurgical Evaluation of Epileptics*, pp 344–351. Berlin: Springer.

Reynolds EH (1967) Effects of folic acid on the mental state and fit frequency of drug treated epileptic patients. *Lancet* **i**: 1086–1088.

Rosental E, Weissman B, Kyllonen K et al (1990) Use of parenteral medium chain triglyceride emulsion for maintaining seizure control in a 5 yr old girl with intractable diarrhoea. *Journal of Parenteral–Enteral Nutrition* **14(5)**: 543–545.

Ross J (1985) *Lang Fu: The Organ Systems of Traditional Chinese Medicine*. Edinburgh: Churchill Livingstone.

Schwartz RH, Bower S & Aynsley Green A (1989a) Metabolic effects of three ketogenic diets in the treatment of severe epilepsy. *Developmental Medicine and Child Neurology* **31**: 152–160.

Schwartz RH, Eaton J, Boyer BD et al (1989b) Ketogenic diets in the treatment of epilepsy: short term clinical effects. *Developmental Medicine and Child Neurology* **31**: 145–151.

Silfvenius H, Olivecrona M, Zetterlund B et al (1989) Paediatric epilepsy surgery. In Nousiaininen U, Riekken P & Aicacsinen E (eds) *Proceedings of the First Woajasalo Epilepsy Symposium*, University of Kuopio, pp 160–163.

Spencer SS (1988) Corpus callosum section and other disconnection procedures for medically intractable epilepsy. *Epilepsia* **29 (supplement 2)**: S85–S99.

Sterman MB (1973) Neurophysiological and clinical studies in sensorimotor EEG, biofeedback training and some effects on epilepsy. In *Biofeedback and Self Control*, pp 363. Chicago: Aldine.

Sterman MB & MacDonald LR (1978) Effects of central cortical EEG training on incidence of poorly controlled seizures. *Epilepsia* **19**: 207–222.

Sterman MB, Wywricta W & Roth SR (1969) Electrophysiological correlates and neural substrates of alimentary behaviour in the cat. *Annals of New York Academy of Science* **157:** 723–739.

Tripp JH, Francis DE, Knight JSA et al (1979) Infant feeding practices—A cause for concern. *British Medical Journal* **2:** 707–709.

Wieser HG (1986) 'Selective amygdalo-hippocampectomy'; indications, investigative technique and results. *Advances and Technical Standards in Neurosurgery* **13:** 39–133.

Wilder RM (1921) The effect of ketonemia on the course of epilepsy. *Mayo Clinical Bulletin* **2:** 307–314.

Williamson PD (1985) Corpus callosum section for intractable epilepsy. Criteria for patient selection. In Reeves AG (ed.) *Epilepsy and the Corpus Callosum*, pp 243–257. New York: Plenum Press.

Wilson PJE (1970) Cerebral hemispherectomy in infantile hemiplegia: a report of 50 cases. *Brain* **93:** 147–180.

Woody RC, Brodie M, Hampton DC et al (1988) Corn oil ketogenic diet for children with intractable seizures. *Journal of Child Neurology* **3:** 21–24.

Woody RC, Steele RW, Knapple WL & Pilkington NS (1989) Impaired phagocytosis in children treated with the ketogenic diet for seizures. *Journal of Pediatrics* **115:** 427–430.

Wurtman RJ (1983) Behavioural effects of nutrients. *Lancet* **i:** 1145–1147.

Wyllie E (1991) Cortical resection for children with epilepsy. *American Journal of Diseases of Children* **145:** 314–320.

6

Febrile seizures

PETER R. CAMFIELD
CAROL S. CAMFIELD

About 8% of people will have a seizure during their life-time (Hauser and Kurland, 1975). One half of these events will be febrile seizures, making this type of seizure the most common convulsive event in the population (Nelson and Ellenberg, 1976; Annegers et al, 1979). Febrile seizures appear to result from the interaction of three factors: fever, susceptible age (generally 6 months to 5 years) and genetic predisposition (which is discussed further in Chapter 3). The child's temperature is usually greater than 38.5°C and the fever may have any cause except CNS infections (Lennox-Buchthal, 1973). The critical age range for febrile seizures suggests a special susceptibility of the maturing nervous system to fever. The genetic tendency has not been fully explored, but it may be transmitted in an autosomal dominant fashion (Tsuboi, 1987; Bethune et al, 1993).

Which child will have a febrile seizure?

Febrile seizures are extremely frightening for families (Baumer et al, 1981). Parents could be educated and prepared if it was clear that their child was at high risk for febrile seizures. No study has been able precisely to identify which newborn will go on to have a febrile seizure; however, a number of factors increase the risk sufficiently that counselling might be warranted for a small group of parents (Forsgren et al, 1991; Bethune et al, 1993).

Bethune and colleagues (1993) carried out a case–control study of 75 children with a first febrile seizure compared with 150 age- and sex-matched controls. In a multivariate analysis, five independent risk factors were noted to predict which child was at risk of a first febrile seizure: (1) a first-degree relative with febrile seizures; (2) a second-degree relative with febrile seizures; (3) delayed neonatal hospital discharge; (4) slow development as judged by parents; and (5) attendance at daycare. Children with none of these risk factors had an estimated 2.2% risk of a febrile seizure. Each one of the factors individually was associated with a 6–11% risk of a first febrile seizure. A child with any two of these factors had a 28% risk of a febrile seizure. It was estimated that 22% of the population has one risk factor, but only 3% of the population will have two or more of these factors. We recommend counselling and anticipatory guidance for families whose

Baillière's Clinical Paediatrics—
Vol. 2, No. 3, August 1994
ISBN 0–7020–1862–7

children have two or more of these risk factors and therefore have at least a 28% chance of an initial febrile seizure.

INITIAL ASSESSMENT OF A CHILD WITH A FEBRILE SEIZURE

Diagnosis

Febrile convulsions typically last only a few minutes and therefore the diagnosis usually has to be based on the history given by the family. The diagnosis is generally straightforward; however, febrile syncope or febrile pallid syncope may sometimes be confused (Stephenson, 1990). Most true febrile seizures have an important rhythmic clonic component. The child's colour is usually normal or flushed at the beginning of the attack, although cyanosis may occur during the seizure. Stephenson (1990) has drawn attention to the clinical details of febrile syncope. In this disorder, the child's colour is usually strikingly pale and the attack begins with limpness followed on occasion by decerebrate posturing and a few myoclonic jerks. The distinction between febrile syncope and febrile convulsions is important. The acute management of the two disorders is similar; however, family counselling about first aid is very different. The risk of epilepsy for a child with pallid syncope is the same as that in the general population, but the risk of recurrent attacks is higher than with febrile seizures.

Lumbar puncture

When a child presents after a febrile seizure, the physician's primary responsibility is to exclude meningitis. Meningitis in a child under 1 year of age may be accompanied by very little nuchal rigidity or other findings of meningeal irritation. The blood white cell count may be normal or low. Therefore, we recommend a lumbar puncture for the majority of children under 1 year of age with a first febrile seizure. For older children there is good evidence that the experienced clinician can accurately diagnose meningitis and therefore routine lumbar puncture is not indicated (Lorber and Sutherland, 1980). Those who are less experienced in the evaluation of the febrile child may have to perform more lumbar punctures.

Blood tests

Routine blood investigations after a febrile seizure have been remarkably unhelpful. Given a clear history in a febrile child of the usual age, there does not appear to be any benefit in laboratory investigation. Blood electrolytes, calcium, glucose and urea levels have all been shown to be of little value (Rutter and Smales, 1977). A complete blood count may give some insight into the cause of fever.

Brain imaging studies

Neuroimaging studies such as computed tomography (CT) or magnetic resonance imaging (MRI) are not indicated after a febrile seizure, even a complicated one (definition below). Nealis et al (1977) have documented that skull radiography does not yield useful information following a febrile seizure. Morales and co-workers (1992) studied CT scans in 44 children with complex febrile seizures and found no significant abnormalities. There is no clinical justification for a systematic study of MRI in children with febrile seizures.

EEG (see also Chapter 8)

There appears to be no benefit from routine EEG in children with febrile seizures. Within 1–2 weeks of a febrile seizure the background activity on the EEG is often abnormal (Frantzen et al, 1968). Possibly more than half of children who have had a febrile seizure will eventually show the particular pattern on EEG of hypnagogic spike and wave as they fall asleep (Doose et al, 1983). Hypnagogic spike and wave is seen most commonly in children of 3 years or older who have had a febrile seizure. In other words, this EEG marker of the febrile seizure tendency appears to emerge at a later age than the peak age for febrile seizures (18 months). There is no explanation at present for this curious observation. The hypnagogic spike and wave pattern is often misinterpreted as being as 'epileptic', but in fact has no long-term significance (Frantzen et al, 1968).

In summary, a history, to establish the diagnosis of febrile seizure, and a physical examination, to find a source of fever and exclude meningitis, are the only investigations that should routinely be undertaken following most febrile seizures.

OUTCOME FOLLOWING A FEBRILE SEIZURE

Death

Several studies have indicated that most parents believed that their child was dying during a febrile seizure (Baumer et al, 1981). This terrifying impression is often most prominent during the postictal phase, when the child is lifeless, with depressed irregular respiration. Death from a febrile seizure has not been described and must be an exceedingly rare event. It is most important that physicians deal with this issue directly in order to help families come to grips with the benign nature of febrile seizures.

Brain damage

Febrile seizures do not cause brain damage. The best evidence for this contention comes from the National Collaborative Perinatal Project (Ellenberg and Nelson, 1978). In the 1950s, this massive American study identified approximately 50 000 children before they were born and followed them until age 7 years. In this cohort, there were 431 sibling pairs discordant for febrile seizures—one child had febrile seizure(s) and the other did not.

At age 7 years, there was no difference in overall intelligence between these siblings, provided the child was neurologically normal before the first febrile seizure.

There is some evidence that a very severe and prolonged febrile seizure may cause brain damage on rare occasions (Aicardi and Chevrie, 1970). The critical duration for a prolonged febrile seizure is unclear, but almost certainly greater than 30 min of continuous seizuring (Meldrum et al, 1974). In our experience the vast majority of children with prolonged febrile seizures longer than 30 min have no neurological sequelae. A similar conclusion was reached by Maytal and Shinnar (1990).

Epilepsy

Children with febrile seizures have at least ten times the risk of developing epilepsy (recurrent afebrile seizures) than children without febrile seizures (Nelson and Ellenberg, 1976; Annegers et al, 1979, 1987; Verity and Golding, 1991). None the less, of all children with febrile seizures 97–98% will not develop epilepsy. It is virtually impossible for the physician to predict accurately whether a given child with a febrile seizure will develop epilepsy at a later date.

Some authors have distinguished between 'simple' or typical febrile seizures (a brief generalized convulsion in an otherwise normal child) and 'complicated', 'complex' or atypical febrile seizures (focal, prolonged or repeated seizures within the same illness) (Duchowny, 1992). It is assumed that simple febrile seizures do not lead to epilepsy while complex seizures frequently do. While intuitively pleasing, this distinction is not very meaningful in an individual child. Some features of the first febrile seizure are statistically predictive of later epilepsy. These risk factors include a complex febrile seizure and neurological or developmental abnormalities (Nelson and Ellenberg, 1976; Annegers et al, 1979). Each one of these risk factors increases the likelihood of epilepsy from 2–3% to about 4–6%. If a child has two or more of these risk factors the chance of subsequent epilepsy is approximately 13% (Nelson and Ellenberg, 1976). In other words, 2% of children with simple febrile seizures later develop epilepsy. Only 13% of children with very complex seizures (two or more risk factors) develop epilepsy; 87% do not. The concept of simple versus complex febrile seizure is statistically correct but not clinically robust.

As mentioned above, the EEG does not predict subsequent epilepsy.

A special concern has been raised about the relationship between prolonged febrile seizures and subsequent intractable complex partial seizures (Rasmussen, 1979). Falconer, a British neurosurgeon, and colleagues (1964) noted that approximately one half of patients who underwent temporal lobectomy for intractable epilepsy had a specific neuropathological abnormality—mesial temporal sclerosis. He noted that 60% of patients with this abnormality had a history of prolonged febrile seizures compared with a much smaller proportion of those without. He hypothesized that the prolonged febrile seizure caused the mesial temporal sclerosis, which in turn led to intractable epilepsy.

Controversy about this hypothesis continues. In the National Collaborative Perinatal Project noted above, none of the children with prolonged febrile seizures developed complex partial seizures by age 7 years (Nelson and Ellenberg, 1976). In addition, in a population-based study of 504 children in the province of Nova Scotia, Canada who developed epilepsy, only two had intractable complex partial seizures following a prolonged febrile seizure with no other aetiology (Camfield et al, 1991). We estimated that the risk of the sequence of a prolonged febrile seizure leading to intractable complex partial seizures occurred no more often than 1 in 75 000 children. This sequence is indeed a rarity.

Severe myoclonic epilepsy of infancy

Clinicians caring for infants with febrile seizure should be aware of this particular epilepsy syndrome (Dravet al, 1985). The children develop normally until 4–6 months of age, when they typically have a first prolonged focal febrile seizure. The children recover well and investigations such as EEG are normal. Repeated prolonged focal febrile seizures follow, often switching sides. In the second year of life, afebrile seizures become more prominent and myoclonus develops. Psychomotor development stagnates. Eventually the EEG shows photosensitive spike and wave abnormalities. This epileptic syndrome is important because the seizures are intractable and the children are virtually always found to be mentally handicapped during long-term follow-up. The reason to emphasize this syndrome in a discussion of febrile seizures is the early presentation of a prolonged focal febrile seizure.

Recurrent febrile seizures

By far the most common sequela of a febrile seizure is a recurrence. Of all children with a first febrile seizure, 30–40% will have a recurrent febrile seizure (Nelson and Ellenberg, 1976; Annegers et al, 1990; Offringa et al, 1992). For those who have had two seizures, again 30–40% will be expected to have an additional febrile seizure.

Two major studies have attempted to identify children with a first febrile seizure who are at high risk of repeated febrile seizures. Knudsen (1985) noted six risk factors identified at the time of the first febrile seizure: age less than 18 months, family history of febrile seizures, family history of epilepsy, developmental delay, complex febrile seizure, attendance at daycare. If a child had none of these factors, the risk of recurrence was 12%. If a child had all of these factors, the recurrence risk was about 80%.

Berg and colleagues (1992) studied 347 children presenting to an emergency room with a first febrile seizure. During a median follow-up of 20 months, 27% had recurrence. There were four factors that predicted recurrence. First was the duration of the fever before the seizure. If a child was recognized to have had a fever for more than 24 h before the seizure, then only 13% recurred. On the other hand, if the fever had been present for only 1 hour before the seizure, 44% recurred. Second, if the child's body temperature was greater than 40°C at the time of the seizure, then only 13% recurred. If the temperature was less than 38.5°C, 35% recurred. In other words, the higher the temperature the less the likelihood of recurrence. Third, if the child was aged less than 18 months at the first febrile seizure, 30% recurred compared with an 18% recurrence rate if the child was older than 18 months. Fourth, a family history of febrile seizures also contributed to the risk of recurrence. With a positive family history, 36% recurred, and without such a history, 20% recurred. Unfortunately, the recurrence risk associated with combinations of these factors was not calculated.

Although these two studies of recurrence after a first febrile seizure differ in some of the identified risk factors, young age and a family history of febrile seizure were found as predictors in both. Others have noted high fever at the time of the seizure to be an important negative predictor (El-Radhi et al, 1986). Therefore, if a child is older than 18 months, has a negative family history of febrile seizures and a temperature of 40°C or more at the time of the seizure, the likelihood of recurrent febrile seizures appears to be very low. On the other hand, a child of less than 18 months with a positive family history of febrile seizures and a febrile seizure at a relatively low body temperature is much more likely to have one or more recurrences.

Attendance at daycare appears to be a risk factor for an initial febrile seizure, as well as for recurrent seizures (Knudsen, 1985; Bethune et al, 1993). The explanation for this association is undoubtedly related to greater exposure to contagious illnesses for children who attend daycare. Because febrile seizures are benign, we do not discourage attendance at daycare for children at risk. Daycare personnel should be taught about the disorder.

MANAGEMENT

Stopping the seizures

There is some evidence that very prolonged febrile seizures, on rare occasions, can damage the brain (Aicardi and Chevrie, 1970). Therefore, it is urgent to stop any febrile seizure still continuing at the time of physician contact. Benzodiazepines appear to be the most effective first-line treatment, especially diazepam. Diazepam is best given at a dose of 0.2 mg/kg intravenously by bolus over 2–3 min. A single dose is effective in about 85% of children with febrile seizures (Knudsen, 1979).

If intravenous access is problematic, diazepam can be given very effectively by rectal administration. The rectal dose is higher at 0.5 mg/kg (Knudsen, 1979). Liquid injectable diazepam is drawn up into an ordinary syringe, the needle removed and the syringe inserted fully into the rectum. The drug can then be delivered as a rapid bolus. Within 4–5 min serum diazepam levels are high (Knudsen, 1977). More than 80% of ongoing febrile seizures are stopped by this method.

In other causes of status epilepticus it is usually recommended to give additional medication with a longer duration of action than diazepam. For febrile seizures this is not often necessary, because it is unusual for such a seizure to start again once it is stopped (Knudsen, 1979). If the seizure stops following administration of diazepam, we would not recommend any further acute treatment.

Antipyretics

When a febrile seizure occurs at home it is not uncommon for families to thrust the child into a cool bath. Such an approach is ill advised. There is no evidence that such a manoeuvre stops febrile seizures and there is concern about precipitating febrile syncope in a susceptible child (Stephenson, 1990).

Antipyretic treatment does not appear to prevent recurrent febrile seizures. We randomized 79 children after a first simple febrile seizure to receive either intensive antipyretic instruction plus a placebo or intensive antipyretic instruction plus daily phenobarbital (Camfield et al, 1980). Over the next year the recurrence rate for those on placebo was 25% compared with 5% for those receiving phenobarbital. This study suggests that very intensive instruction about the use of antipyretics does not alter the recurrence rate for febrile seizures.

Many authorities have suggested sponging a febrile child in cool water to reduce fever rapidly and prevent recurrent febrile seizures. Newman (1985) randomized 137 children with an average age of 1 year and a temperature of 39 °C or greater to receive oral antipyretic medication plus 20 min sponging in tepid water or antipyretics only: 30 and 50 min later there was no advantage to sponging. Sponging as a method of temperature control should be abandoned.

Because families are very upset by febrile seizures, and because they realize that fever is an essential ingredient in recurrent febrile seizures, they are prone to become 'fever phobic' (Schmitt, 1980). Given the above evidence, it is important that they come to understand that it is virtually impossible to prevent a recurrence by attempting to control the child's temperature.

Medication treatment

Daily prophylactic medication

After one or more febrile seizures daily, valproic acid or daily phenobarbital may be effective to prevent recurrence (Wolf et al, 1977; Camfield et al, 1980; Herranc et al, 1984). Compliance with daily medication is often unsatisfactory and several large studies of daily phenobarbital have suggested that it is not overwhelmingly successful (Newton, 1988; Farwell et al, 1990). Daily phenytoin or carbamazepine are not effective in the prevention of recurrent febrile seizures (Bacon et al, 1981; Camfield et al, 1982; Anthony and Hawke, 1983).

The potential utility of daily prophylactic medication to prevent recurrent seizures must be balanced against the possible side-effects. There is a danger of fatal hepatic failure from valproic acid (Dreifus et al, 1987). Several studies have suggested that phenobarbital may cause cognitive deficits in children (Camfield et al, 1979; Farwell et al, 1990). Since febrile seizures are benign, we conclude that there is virtually no indication for daily prophylactic medication in the treatment of febrile seizures.

Rectal diazepam at the time of fever

Knudsen and Vestermark (1978) compared daily phenobarbital prophylaxis with rectal diazepam 0.5 mg/kg given every 12 h at the time of fever. Both treatments were equally effective. Rectal diazepam at the time of fever certainly limits the child's drug exposure but may be ineffective in 15–20% of patients for whom the seizure is the first indication of the fever. None the less, this approach may be reasonable for a selected group of extremely anxious families, provided the child has few caretakers. Intermittent rectal diazepam does cause some degree of sedation and the long-term side-effects of benzodiazepine use in toddlers have not been studied.

Home rectal diazepam at the time of a seizure

Based on the premise that the only dangerous febrile seizure is a very prolonged seizure, then it is reasonable to teach some families to give rectal diazepam only at the time of a seizure. Although there have been no randomized trials of this approach, it is clear that rectal diazepam can be successfully administered by families (Hoppu and Santavuori, 1981; Camfield et al, 1989).

Criteria for selecting families to learn how to use rectal diazepam are not clear-cut. The child must have few caretakers and families must understand the technique. Some children who are candidates for home rectal diazepam administration are those with poor access to medical care and those with extremely anxious parents. An initial prolonged febrile seizure is not a firm indication because the risk is less than 2% for a second prolonged febrile seizure (Nelson and Ellenberg, 1978).

Because doses of rectal diazepam higher than 0.5 mg/kg may cause severe respiratory depression, families must be carefully taught how to administer this medication (Hoppu and Santavuori, 1981). The child should receive a test dose under direct medical supervision to ensure there are no untoward effects.

Early in our own experience with home rectal diazepam, we learned that families tended to teach other family members how to give the rectal diazepam (Camfield et al, 1989). We now insist that all the teaching be done in a paediatric centre.

Oral diazepam at the time of fever

Currently, there are two published controlled studies of the use of oral diazepam at the time of fever to prevent recurrent febrile seizures. One of these studies found oral intermittent diazepam to be ineffective (Autret et al, 1990). A larger American study randomized 406 children after at least one febrile seizure to oral diazepam (0.33 mg/kg per dose every 8 h) at the time of even the slightest fever or to placebo (Rossman et al, 1993). After 36 months the recurrence rate for those receiving diazepam was 22% compared with 31% for those taking placebo. This modest reduction was balanced by a 40% incidence of moderate diazepam side-effects. There would seem to be little benefit from oral diazepam for most children after a first febrile seizure.

Dealing with parents' anxiety

The most important issue in febrile seizure management is family counsel-ling. If families truly understand the benign nature of febrile seizures, additional treatment is not needed. In our institution if a child has had a febrile seizure, the parents see an educational slide–tape show about febrile seizures and receive a written hand-out (Appendix; Camfield et al, 1981). Families appear to retain the factual information.

The physician must deal directly with the parent's fear that their child nearly died during the seizure. Issues related to fever phobia must be discussed. We recommend a follow-up visit with the physician several weeks after the seizure to review the factual information and to be sure that life has returned to normal.

SUMMARY

There is convincing evidence that febrile seizures are benign, do not injure the brain and are only rarely precursors of epilepsy. There is no evidence that prevention of febrile seizures can prevent epilepsy.

The investigation of a child with febrile seizure is primarily that of a history and physical examination with a lumbar puncture to exclude meningitis in selected patients. There is no need for more complex investigation.

The treatment for most children with a febrile seizure is reassurance. On rare occasions, the family may be taught the use of rectal diazepam for home use at the time of a recurrent febrile seizure, but otherwise antiepileptic medication is not warranted.

APPENDIX: WHAT PARENTS SHOULD KNOW ABOUT FEVER AND SEIZURES

Babies and young children often have illnesses that are accompanied by fever. Most children with fever suffer only minor discomfort that can be relieved by paracetamol. In about 3–4% of infants and toddlers, however, fever brings on a seizure at some time during childhood.

These kinds of seizures are not harmful to the child and do not cause brain damage. They are, however, quite upsetting to parents. These questions and answers should help you cope if your child ever has a febrile seizure.

What is a febrile seizure?

A febrile seizure is a convulsion or fit brought on by an elevated temperature. During a febrile seizure, the child usually loses consciousness. The muscles may stiffen or jerk. The seizure may last for several minutes. Then the movements stop, and the child regains consciousness—but may be a little groggy afterwards.

Does it happen to many children?

Yes. Febrile seizures are very common. One in 25 children has a febrile seizure at one time or another, usually between the ages of 6 months and 4 years.

If my child has a febrile seizure, does that mean she has epilepsy?

No. Epilepsy is a disorder of repeated seizures that occur *without* fever.

Will febrile seizures cause epilepsy or brain damage?

No. No matter how dramatic and frightening febrile seizures may appear, they do not cause brain damage or epilepsy. Even very prolonged seizures lasting an hour or more almost never cause harm. Studies show that 97% of all children with febrile seizures do *not* have epilepsy later on. The odds are overwhelming that a child who has febrile seizures will be normal.

If my child has one febrile seizure, will it happen again?

Realistically, for many children the answer is Yes. Almost one half of children who have had a first febrile seizure will have one or more recurrences. Even repeated febrile seizures, however, do not mean that a child has epilepsy. Your child will outgrow the tendency to have febrile seizures as he or she approaches 3–4 years of age.

What can parents do during a seizure?

There is nothing you can do to make the seizure stop. The most important thing is to stay calm. Place your child on a soft surface, lying on his or her side or abdomen. Do not restrain the child, and do not put anything in their mouth. Your child will not choke.

Try to observe exactly what happens, so that you can describe it later, and time how long the seizure lasts. If the seizure stops in less than 10 minutes, there is no urgent rush to get medical attention. Call to tell us what has happened, and make an appointment to bring the child in for an examination.

If the seizure lasts more than 10 minutes, take your child right away to the nearest doctor or hospital where medication to stop the seizure can be given. Drive very carefully. A few minutes longer will not make any important difference.

Can we do anything to prevent a seizure?

No. Constant worry about your child's temperature will only upset you and will not prevent seizures. In some children, a seizure is the first indication that a child has a fever. Lowering your child's fever with paracetamol may make him or her more comfortable but will not ward off a seizure. Ask us about the right dose to use. Don't use sponge baths or fans to lower the child's temperature. These measures only make a sick child more uncomfortable and do not prevent seizures.

Only a few special children need long-term daily medication to prevent febrile seizures. If we feel medication might be indicated for your child, we can discuss it together.

Once the seizure is over, does our child need special treatment?

Your child may be a little cranky for a day or so, but this will pass. Resume your usual routines. Put your child to sleep at the usual time, in his or her own bed. Don't worry about whether you will hear a seizure; a bed or crib is a safe place for a seizure, and if the next one is so brief that you don't wake up, then no intervention was needed.

Can a child who has febrile seizures lead a normal life?

Yes, if you allow it. Your child hasn't changed, and there is no need for you to change your life-style or your relationship with your child. Just make sure your child has the love, security and discipline that every child needs.

REFERENCES

Aicardi J & Chevrie JJ (1970) Convulsive status epilepticus in infants and children. *Epilepsia* **11:** 187–197.

Annegers JF, Hauser WA, Elveback LR et al (1979) The risk of epilepsy following febrile convulsions. *Neurology* **29:** 297–303.

Annegers JF, Hauser WA, Shirto S et al (1987) Factors prognostic of unprovoked seizures after febrile convulsions. *New England Journal of Medicine* **316:** 493–498.

Annegers JF, Blakely SA, Hauser WA et al (1990) Recurrence of febrile convulsions in a population-based cohort. *Epilepsy Research* **5:** 209–216.

Anthony J & Hawke S (1983) Phenobarbital compared with carbamazepine in prevention of recurrent febrile convulsions. *American Journal of Diseases of Children* **137:** 892–895.

Autret E, Billard C, Bertrand P et al (1990) Double-blind randomized trial of diazepam versus placebo for prevention of recurrence of febrile seizures. *Journal of Pediatrics* **117:** 490–495.

Bacon C, Mucklow J, Rawlins M et al (1981) Placebo-controlled study of phenobarbitone and phenytoin in the prophylaxis of febrile convulsions. *Lancet* **ii:** 600–603.

Baumer JH, David TJ, Valentine SJ et al (1981) Many parents think their child is dying when having a first febrile convulsion. *Developmental Medicine and Child Neurology* **23:** 462–464.

Berg AT, Shinnar S, Hauser WA et al (1992) Predictors of recurrent febrile seizures: a prospective study of the circumstances surrounding the initial febrile seizure. *New England Journal of Medicine* **327:** 1112–1127.

Bethune P, Gordon KG, Dooley JM et al (1993) Which child will have a febrile seizure? *American Journal of Diseases of Children* **147:** 35–39.

Camfield CS, Chaplin S, Doyle AB et al (1979) Side effects of phenobarbital in toddlers: behavioral and cognitive aspects. *Journal of Pediatrics* **95:** 361–365.

Camfield CS, Camfield PR, Smith E & Dooley JM (1989) Home use of rectal diazepam to prevent status epilepticus in children with convulsive disorders. *Journal of Child Neurology* **4:** 125–126.

Camfield CS, Camfield PR, Dooley JM & Gordon K (1991) What type of afebrile seizures are preceded by febrile seizures? A population based study in children. *Epilepsia* **32:** 439 (abstract).

Camfield PR, Camfield CS, Shapiro S et al (1980) The first febrile seizure—antipyretic instruction plus either phenobarbital or placebo to prevent a recurrence. *Journal of Pediatrics* **97:** 16–21.

Camfield PR, Camfield CS, Buchholz K et al (1981) Information on febrile seizures for parents and caretakers. In Nelson K & Ellenberg J (eds) *Febrile Seizures*, pp 245–252. New York: Raven Press.

Camfield PR, Camfield CS & Tibbles JAR (1982) Carbamazepine does not prevent febrile seizures in phenobarbital failures. *Neurology* **32:** 288–299.

Doose H, Ritter K & Volzke E (1983) EEG longitudinal studies in febrile convulsions, genetic aspects. *Neuropediatrics* **14:** 81–87.

Dravet C, Bureau M & Roger J (1985) Benign myoclonic epilepsy in infants. In Roger J, Dravet C, Bureau M et al (eds) *Epileptic Syndromes in Infancy, Childhood and Adolescence*, pp 58–67. London: John Libbey Eurotext.

Dreifus FE, Santilli N, Langer DH et al (1987) Valproic acid hepatic fatalities: a retrospective review. *Neurology* **37:** 379–385.

Duchowny M (1992) Febrile seizures in childhood. In Wyllie E (ed.) *Epilepsy: Principles and Practice*, pp 647–653. Philadelphia: Lea and Febiger.

Ellenberg JH & Nelson KB (1978) Febrile seizures and later intellectual performance. *Archives of Neurology* **35:** 17–21.

El-Radhi AS, Withana K & Banejeh S (1986) Recurrence rate of febrile convulsions related to the degree of pyrexia during the first attack. *Clinical Pediatrics* **25**: 311–313.

Falconer MA, Serafetinides EA & Corsellis JA (1964) Etiology and pathogenesis of temporal lobe epilepsy. *Archives of Neurology* **10**: 233–248.

Farwell J, Lee YJ, Hirtz DG et al (1990) Phenobarbital for febrile seizures—effects on intelligence and on seizure recurrence. *New England Journal of Medicine* **322**: 364–369.

Forsgren L, Sidenvall R, Blomquist H et al (1991) Pre- and perinatal factors in febrile convulsions. *Acta Paediatrica Scandinavica* **80**: 218–225.

Frantzen E, Lennox-Buchthal M, Nygaard A & Stene J (1968) Longitudinal EEG and clinical study of children with febrile convulsions. *Electroencephalography and Clinical Neurophysiology* **24**: 197–212.

Hauser WA & Kurland LT (1975) The epidemiology of epilepsy in Rochester, Minnesota, 1935 through 1967. *Epilepsia* **16**: 1–66.

Herranc J, Armijo J & Arteaga R (1984) Effectiveness and toxicity of phenobarbital, primidone, and sodium valproate in the prevention of febrile convulsions. *Epilepsia* **25**: 89–95.

Hoppu K & Santavuori P (1981) Diazepam rectal solution for home treatment of acute seizures. *Acta Paediatrica Scandinavica* **70**: 369–372.

Knudsen FU (1977) Plasma diazepam in infants after rectal administration in solution and by suppository. *Acta Paediatrica Scandinavica* **66**: 563–567.

Knudsen FU (1979) Rectal administration of diazepam in solution in the acute treatment of convulsions in infants and children. *Archives of Disease in Childhood* **54**: 855–857.

Knudsen FU (1985) Recurrence risk after first febrile seizure and effect of short term diazepam prophylaxis. *Archives of Disease in Childhood* **60**: 1045–1049.

Knudsen FU & Vestermark S (1978) Prophylactic diazepam or phenobarbitone in febrile convulsions: a prospective, controlled study. *Archives of Disease in Childhood* **53**: 660–663.

Lennox-Buchthal MA (1973) Febrile convulsions. A reappraisal. *Electroencephalography and Clinical Neurophysiology* (**supplement 32**): 1–132.

Lorber J & Sunderland R (1980) Lumbar puncture in children with convulsions associated with fever. *Lancet* **i**: 785–786.

Maytal J & Shinnar S (1990) Febrile status epilepticus. *Pediatrics* **86**: 611–616.

Meldrum BS, Horton RW & Brierley JB (1974) Epileptic brain damage in adolescent baboons following seizures induced by allylglycine. *Brain* **97**: 407–418.

Morales A, Bass N, Lake-Smith K et al (1992) Computerized tomographs and febrile seizures. *Annals of Neurology* **32**: 432 (abstract).

Nealis JGT, McFadden SW, Asnes RA et al (1977) Routine skull roentgenograms in the management of simple febrile seizures. *Journal of Pediatrics* **90**: 595–596.

Nelson KB & Ellenberg JH (1976) Predictors of epilepsy in children who have experienced febrile seizures. *New England Journal of Medicine* **295**: 1029–1033.

Nelson KB & Ellenberg JH (1978) Prognosis in children with febrile seizures. *Pediatrics* **61**: 720–727.

Newman J (1985) Evaluation of sponging to reduce body temperature in febrile children. *Canadian Medical Association Journal* **132**: 641–642.

Newton RW (1988) Randomized controlled trials of phenobarbitone and valproate in febrile convulsions. *Archives of Disease in Childhood* **63**: 1189–1192.

Offringa M, Derksen-Lubsen G, Bossuyt PM & Lubsen J (1992) Seizure recurrence after a first febrile seizure: a multivariate approach. *Developmental Medicine and Child Neurology* **34**: 15–24.

Rasmussen T (1979) Relative significance of isolated infantile convulsions as a primary cause of focal epilepsy. *Epilepsia* **20**: 395–401.

Rossman NP, Colton T, Labazzo RNC et al (1993) A controlled trial of diazepam administered during febrile illnesses to prevent recurrence of febrile seizures. *New England Journal of Medicine* **329**: 79–84.

Rutter N & Smales ORC (1977) Role of routine investigations in children presenting with their first febrile convulsion. *Archives of Disease in Childhood* **52**: 188–191.

Schmitt BD (1980) Fever phobia. *American Journal of Diseases of Children* **134**: 176–181.

Stephenson JBP (1990) *Fits and Faints*. Oxford: MacKeith Press.

Tsuboi T (1987) Genetic analysis of febrile convulsions. *Human Genetics* **75**: 7–14.

Verity CM & Golding J (1991) Risk of epilepsy after febrile convulsions: a national cohort study. *British Medical Journal* **303:** 1373–1376.

Wolf CM, Carr A, David DC et al (1977) The value of phenobarbital in the child who has had a single febrile seizure: a controlled prospective study. *Pediatrics* **59:** 378–385.

7

Epilepsy, education and the role of mental handicap

FRANK M. C. BESAG

Misconceptions about the role of epilepsy in education abound. The contrasting assumptions that epilepsy always has a major effect on education or that epilepsy seldom affects school performance are equally wrong. Although many children with epilepsy have no educational problems, a large proportion do encounter difficulties. An understanding of the problems that might arise enables early intervention and the possibility of minimizing any disruption to the child's education.

This chapter is in five main sections. In the first section the literature on epilepsy and education is reviewed. In the second, the causes of educational failure in the child with epilepsy are examined. Most of these causes apply in children with or without mental handicap. The relationships between epilepsy and mental handicap are discussed in the third section. The conflicting literature on so-called 'cognitive deterioration' in children with epilepsy is reviewed and the results from the St Piers Lingfield studies, carried out over the past seven decades, are summarized. The concepts of cognitive arrest or slowing, in contrast to cognitive deterioration, are highlighted. Epilepsy as a cause and as a consequence of brain dysfunction and deterioration are distinguished. The fourth section covers the important topics of diagnosis, assessment, investigation and management of children with epilepsy and learning disability. The role of special schools for children with epilepsy is covered in the fifth section.

EPILEPSY AND EDUCATION

The long history of prejudice against children with epilepsy has led to a well-intentioned counter-reaction encouraging the attitude that all children with epilepsy are capable of coping well with normal education. The only satisfactory way of resolving the questions surrounding education in children with epilepsy is to carry out careful epidemiological studies. There have been a number of attempts to carry out such studies. All of them have shown unequivocally that children with epilepsy are more likely to encounter educational difficulty, although the details of the studies show some variability.

Baillière's Clinical Paediatrics—
Vol. 2, No. 3, August 1994
ISBN 0–7020–1862–7

Pond and Bidwell (1960) surveyed patients with epilepsy in 14 general practices. One third of the children of school age (14 of 39 children) were identified as having some difficulties in education, especially as a result of behavioural disorders. Although the publication by Ounsted et al (1966) was based on a somewhat selected sample, it emphasized the point that a high proportion of children with temporal lobe epilepsy had poor academic achievement, even if they were of normal overall intelligence. The classic Isle of Wight study (Rutter et al, 1970) found an excess of reading retardation of 2 years or more in children with epilepsy, even if they were of normal or above-normal intelligence. This work is still widely quoted because it was a true epidemiological study examining all the children around 10 years of age in a defined geographical location.

Although earlier papers had pointed to the suggestion that children with epilepsy might encounter intellectual difficulties, as discussed in the section below on mental handicap, these were generally based on selected populations, allowing no general conclusions to be drawn. The widely quoted Green and Hartlage (1971) paper falls into this category; the 50 children and adolescents all attended an outpatient epilepsy clinic at Indiana University Medical Center and consequently were a selected population. The publication by Holdsworth and Whitmore (1974a) to some extent redressed the balance. This was not a study based on an entire childhood population, because it excluded children attending special schools. However, the results are of particular interest because the authors attempted to locate all the children attending ordinary schools in a particular area.

Eighty-five children with epilepsy fulfilled their criteria of attendance at an ordinary school and having had a seizure during the prior 12 months (52 children) or being treated with antiepileptic drugs over that period (33 children). The relatively low prevalence figures obtained by the study, namely 1.6 per 1000 in the primary schools and 2.4 per 1000 in the secondary schools, probably reflect the fact that additional cases were excluded because they were not attending ordinary schools. They were able to classify 64 of the children into three groups, based on their educational perform-ance. Twenty children (31%) were maintaining an average to a superior level of performance, 34 (53%) were 'holding their own at a below-average level' and 10 (16%) were seriously behind.

The data presented did not suggest that poor attendance was the cause of the educational difficulties. The teaching staff were asked to assess atten-tiveness and behaviour. Because the evaluation was not carried out in a blinded fashion using standardized tests, the results might reflect a degree of observer bias. Nevertheless, it is interesting that 42% of the children were noted to have problems with attention and were described in terms such as listless, lethargic, dull, apathetic and 'just not with us'. Absence seizures were unlikely to account for the descriptions, since only four children had these. Twenty-one per cent were said to have had 'noticeably deviant behaviour'. Fourteen of these 18 children were described as aggressive, attention-seeking, objectionable, truculent, spiteful or bullying. Two were truants and four were isolated or withdrawn. Among those who were failing in school there were more boys than girls, and more of these children had major seizures.

A surprising finding of the study was a statistically significant result that children whose behaviour was not causing concern were twice as likely to be taking phenobarbitone. This finding is in sharp contrast to the personal experience of many paediatricians who have found that phenobarbitone can be associated with gross behavioural disturbance. The frequency of the seizures seemed to have no bearing on educational outcome or poor attendance. In keeping with other studies, however, they found that three of the four children with absence seizures alone were progressing well. Behavioural disturbance was associated both with poor educational performance and with the occurrence of seizures. The authors decried the fact that it was exceptional to find 'co-operation between doctor, psychologist and teachers in the management of the 32 children who presented problems with frequent seizures, poor educational outcome and behavioural difficulties'. These comments were supported in a second paper by the same authors (Holdsworth and Whitmore, 1947b).

A survey of Cesena, Italy, and the surrounding villages carried out by Pazzaglia and Frank-Pazzaglia (1976) identified 38 children with epilepsy out of a total population of 13 000 school-age children aged 6–14 years. They found a prevalence of about 3 per 1000, suggesting that they located a large proportion of the children with elilepsy. Their results reinforced the findings of earlier studies in showing a large proportion of children with educational difficulty and other problems. Of the 38 children, 27 were of normal intelligence and 11 (29%) were 'retarded', which they defined as having an IQ of less than 80, although 10 of the 11 children had an IQ lower than 70. They commented that 24 of the 27 children of normal intelligence had what they described as 'chronic depressive syndromes' with feelings of inferiority, insecurity and a tendency to give up and withdraw. About half the children had a normal record in school. Seven (18%) were behind their grade in school and 13 (34%) were in special schools.

Another outstanding finding of the Pazzaglia and Frank-Pazzaglia study was the unsatisfactory attitudes of teachers and parents of other pupils in the class. All the teachers felt they had no training and most were unwilling to teach pupils with epilepsy. The positive recommendation was that the teachers suggested pupils with epilepsy should be taught in normal classes on the condition that there be close collaboration with a team of physicians and psychologists. Five per cent of the teachers thought that all pupils with epilepsy should be taught in special classes.

Provided the pupils did not have major seizures at school, problems tended not to arise. Of the eight pupils who had major seizures at school the classmates were anxious and the parents afraid that their own children might be damaged psychologically by seeing a seizure. In some cases they tried to have the child with epilepsy removed from the class.

Stores and co-workers published a series of papers discussing educational difficulties of children with epilepsy (Stores, 1971, 1973, 1975, 1978, 1981, 1989; Stores and Hart, 1976; Stores et al, 1978).

Stores and Hart (1976) examined reading skills in children with generalized epileptiform discharges and focal discharges. Seventeen children (ten boys and seven girls) with generalized discharges were matched for age and sex with 17 who had persistent focal discharges on either side and with children who did not have epilepsy. They found no difference between the reading skills of children who had electrographically generalized epilepsy with 'subclinical seizure discharge' and those of matched controls who did not have epilepsy. However, children with persistent focal spike discharges tended to have a lower reading level than matched controls, especially with regard to reading accuracy. These changes were largely the effect of left hemisphere focal spikes. The reading skills of boys with epilepsy, whatever the type, were worse than those of girls with epilepsy. This sex difference was not found in the control children who did not have epilepsy.

Stores and colleagues (1978) applied a number of measures of inattentiveness to 36 boys and 35 girls with epilepsy. The boys were significantly worse than the girls. No such sex difference was seen in any of the measures amongst children who did not have epilepsy. The results were of particular interest with regard to the distractibility test: the distraction applied to children who did not have epilepsy lowered the scores, as expected, but performance improved in those who did have epilepsy, suggesting that these children were in some way under-aroused and derived benefit from the alerting effect of the noise. The other point of particular interest was that children with the three per second spike-and-wave EEG pattern, typical of absence seizures, were significantly *less* impaired on vigilance and distractibility tests than other subgroups.

The study on behavioural disorder (Stores, 1977) again showed a striking difference between boys and girls with epilepsy. In the control group, without epilepsy, the boys did not differ greatly in terms of behavioural disturbance from the girls, but the boys with epilepsy were characterized particularly by anxiety, inattentiveness and social isolation. The group with left temporal spike discharges were the most disturbed and were significantly more overactive than boys who did not have epilepsy.

In the fourth study, reported by Stores et al (1978), the dependency of children with epilepsy was examined. The results were based on the Self-Administered Dependency Questionnaire (SADQ) assessing four types of dependency: affection, communication, assistance and travel. Clear sex differences were seen. The boys of primary school age with epilepsy showed a significantly greater need for affection and the presence of their mother compared with boys of the same age who did not have epilepsy. Boys of secondary school age (11–18 years) were significantly more in need of practical help. The girls with epilepsy, however, were not significantly more dependent than girls who did not have epilepsy. Both boys and girls with persistent left temporal spike discharges had significantly greater need for physical emotional contact with their mothers than either children with generalized epilepsy or those with a persistent right temporal discharge.

Stores has emphasized that, although some children with epilepsy have more educational problems in terms of learning and behaviour than other children, many have no such difficulties. He has underlined the importance of identifying those who had such problems and offering early intervention.

He also concluded that boys were much more vulnerable than girls to behavioural problems. The other main conclusions related to the importance of persistent left temporal spike discharges, which seemed to be associated with reading retardation, inattentiveness, emotional dependence and, in boys, other types of disturbed behaviour, especially overactivity.

In summary, Stores and co-workers have made an important contribution to the understanding of the difficulties that are likely to occur in the education of children with epilepsy, drawing particular attention to the vulnerability of boys with left temporal discharges.

The papers based on the National Child Development Study are also of particular merit because this was a very carefully conducted epidemiological investigation of a cohort of 17 733 children born in the week 3–9 March 1958 in England, Scotland and Wales. A total of 15 496 of the original children were traced and alive at 11 years of age when the epilepsy prevalence was 4.1 per 1000. This figure suggests that, in contrast to some of the previously reported studies, few, if any, cases were missed. The criteria for inclusion were strict. At 11 years of age there were 346 possible cases of epilepsy but the diagnosis was firmly established in only 64. Of these cases, 22 (34%) were in special education by the age of 16 years. These studies again showed that those remaining in mainstream schooling tended to have primary generalized epilepsy and the majority had well-controlled seizures. However, even those children who did remain within mainstream school tended to have lower reading and mathematics scores than the general age-matched population. Most of the children who were in special education were placed there because of intellectual impairment rather than severity of their epilepsy. This excellent epidemiological study has been reported by Ross et al (1980), Verity and Ross (1985) and Kurtz et al (1987).

A further epidemiological study of interest was performed by Ellenberg et al (1985) as part of the National Collaborative Perinatal Project of the National Institute of Neurological and Communicative Disorders and Stroke (NCPP) in the USA. The NCPP followed the outcome of the 54 000 pregnancies in 1959. Ellenberg and co-workers identified 518 children who had one or more non-febrile seizure after the newborn period; 368 of these underwent intelligence testing at 7 years. Ninety-eight children with non-febrile seizures had at least one sibling in the study. By using sibling controls, the authors concluded that, although the mean IQ score of 91.5 was less than that of the general population, it was not significantly different from that of sibling controls. Nevertheless, their study would imply poorer intellectual performance of children with epilepsy, compared with the general population. This paper is discussed further in the section on epilepsy and mental handicap.

One of the outstanding workers in the field of epidemiology is Sillanpää in Finland, who has published a number of papers. One of the more recent publications (Sillanpää, 1992) reports results obtained from 143 children with epilepsy out of a population of 21 104 children aged 4–15 years. He commented that the most frequent neurological impairments were mental retardation (31.4%), speech disorders (27.5%) and specific learning disorders (23.1%). He concluded that there was a 22-fold risk of occurrence of a handicap in children with epilepsy compared with controls. In earlier reviews (Sillanpää, 1983, 1990) he concluded that 27.5% of children with epilepsy did not complete their basic education or required schooling in establishments for learning disability.

The consensus from these studies is that, although the educational progress of some children with epilepsy is in the normal or superior range, a large proportion have a degree of educational difficulty. The precise figures depend on the ability to locate and include all cases, and on the operational definition of educational difficulty. In broad terms it appears that between one quarter and one half of all children with epilepsy experience a degree of educational difficulty. Up to one quarter may need special schooling of one type or another. The role of the epilepsy special schools, which are required for less than 1% of children with epilepsy, is discussed in the final section of this chapter.

CAUSES OF EDUCATIONAL FAILURE IN THE CHILD WITH EPILEPSY

The present author has attempted to classify causes of learning disability and behavioural disturbance in children with epilepsy (Besag et al, 1989b; Besag, 1993). By affecting learning and behaviour, these factors may lead to educational failure. The suggested classifications are shown in Table 1. This

Table 1. Factors that may affect learning and behaviour in a subject with epilepsy.

The epilepsy itself
  Prodrome
  Aura
  Automatism
  Postictal changes
  Interictal psychoses
  Focal discharges
  Frequent absence seizures
Treatment of the epilepsy
Reactions to the epilepsy
Associated brain damage
Causes that are equally applicable to those without epilepsy

review was not comprehensive but was intended to indicate that a rational classification of the causes of educational difficulty in a child with epilepsy can facilitate rational and appropriate management. Failure to classify the cause of the learning or behavioural disturbance correctly can lead to mismanagement. An area that was not covered adequately in the earlier review by the present author was the effect of sleep disturbance on learning and behaviour. Stores (1990) has recently emphasized the need for examining sleep disturbance in this context.

The epilepsy itself

Prodrome

Some people experience changes in mood for hours or days before a seizure. These experiences are likely to affect both learning and behaviour. It would be quite inappropriate for the school teacher to admonish or punish the child for being mildly irritable during this period. Although the need for discipline remains, the way in which it is administered needs to be moderated at this time by an understanding of the organic nature of the mood disturbance.

Aura

A focal discharge in the brain, typically in the temporal lobe although sometimes elsewhere, may cause sensory phenomena that are, strictly speaking, simple partial seizures. Auras typically last for a few seconds. The most classical auras are unpleasant sensations in the epigastrium, odd smells or flashing lights. The dysphoric aura may be described as intensely unpleasant and quite unlike anything else. Children experiencing multiple auras may find these much more distressing than full-blown seizures, since auras occur in full consciousness and are usually remembered. The child may think that this is a sign of madness and may be unwilling to let others know of the experience. Because auras can also herald full-blown seizures they may, understandably, be associated with anxiety. All these factors are likely to lead to problems if auras occur in the classroom, particularly if teachers do not understand why the child appears distressed and adopt a punitive approach. The many varieties of aura, usually unpleasant but occasionally pleasant, are well described in the literature; see, for example, O'Donohoe's book *Epilepsies of Childhood* (1994).

Automatism

Various types of automatism are well described in classical papers (e.g. Knox, 1968). Fenton (1972) has given one of the most widely accepted definitions: 'A state of clouding of consciousness, which occurs during or immediately after a seizure and during which the individual retains control of posture and muscle tone but performs simple or complex movements and actions without being aware of what is happening'. Automatisms occurring after an obvious tonic–clonic seizure may be more readily accepted than those occurring as a result of a complex partial seizure, since the latter may not be recognized as being a seizure at all. Because these behaviours, which can sometimes appear quite bizarre, may be open to misinterpretation by teachers and may be the butt of teasing by classmates, they may have a profound educational implication.

Postictal changes

Sleepiness is the most common postictal change. If the child needs to sleep for long periods after a seizure this may be very disruptive to schooling.

Other types of postictal change vary from subtle to the florid; these can include postictal depressive, manic and schizophreniform paranoid changes. Such changes are usually short-lived, perhaps lasting a few days; they do not necessarily require treatment, but certainly require great support and understanding. Severe postictal psychoses are uncommon but may need emergency treatment.

Fugue states

These are again rare but can easily be misinterpreted. The definition of a fugue comprises wandering, apparently impaired awareness and subsequent amnesia for the events during the fugue. Although the literature leaves some doubt about the existence of epilepsy-related fugues (e.g. Lishman, 1978), the present author is in no doubt about this phenomenon and has recorded several, unpublished, cases of postictal fugue. Fugues may be misdiagnosed as psychiatric disorders arising out of relationship problems when they are nothing of the sort. Improving the antiepileptic therapy may resolve the problem. Ictal fugues are particularly rare and are generally associated with complex partial seizure status epilepticus.

Interictal psychoses

These are not usually seen in children but may certainly be seen in adolescents. The present author has seen interictal psychoses in several teenagers. They may last for several months and, if severe, may impair education to a major degree until they resolve or are treated satisfactorily.

Focal discharges

The association between deficits in reading skills and focal spike discharges in either the left temporal lobe or the immediately adjacent area was emphasized by Stores (1978). Several studies have suggested an association between left temporal discharges and behavioural disturbance. The importance of behavioural disturbance in disrupting education is all too evident and has been documented in reviews, including that of Pazzaglia and Frank-Pazzaglia (1976). Binnie (1980) highlighted the importance of focal epileptiform discharges in causing transitory cognitive impairment. In a more recent study by Marston et al (1993), attempts were made to determine the psychosocial effects of transitory cognitive impairment in children attending a special school. Although there were some confounding factors in this study it appears that the suppression of discharges leading to transitory cognitive impairment improved overall psychosocial performance. The role of frontal lobe discharges has probably been underemphasized. The present author's experience suggests that frequent frontal discharges may affect behaviour and learning to a major degree. Further systematic study of this phenomenon is required.

All these results point to the importance of carefully planned EEG investigation of children who may have abnormal EEG discharges and who are failing educationally. Without accurate information, rational intervention cannot be planned. In particular, if the doctor does now know that the abnormal discharges are there, they are unlikely to be treated.

Frequent absence seizures

The favourable prognosis, in educational terms, of children with absence seizures is not what might be expected: it would be plausible to think that frequent subtle interruptions of awareness in the classroom might have a profound effect on school performance. The good educational prognosis is almost certainly the consequence of the fact that typical absence seizures tend not to be associated with other forms of brain dysfunction, often occurring in children of normal intelligence. For example, Holdsworth and Whitmore (1974a) identified four children with absence seizures, three of whom were average to superior in their level of performance. Pure typical absence seizures are relatively uncommon, probably accounting for less than 5% of cases of childhood epilepsy. Although most children with occasional typical absence seizures progress well, some who have very frequent absence seizures may encounter considerable difficulties. The group with atypical absences often have EEG patterns that differ from the classical three per second spike-and-wave pattern of typical absence seizures. The abnormalities include polyspike and wave, or slow spike and wave. The discharges may be of varying morphology and are sometimes associated with the Lennox–Gastaut syndrome. The present author has shown, with the help of specialized monitoring developed at St Piers Lingfield, that spike-and-wave discharges may occur thousands of times per day. In the small number of children who have such frequent epileptiform discharges, educational progress and social interaction are clearly hampered to a major degree. Although the manifestations of the discharges may vary widely from one child to another, it seems that impairment of the educational abilities while they are occurring is almost inevitable.

Non-convulsive status epilepticus

If the epileptiform discharges are generalized, non-convulsive status epilepticus may represent an extreme form of the frequent absence seizures described above. Non-convulsive status epilepticus may also result from prolonged complex partial seizures. This subject has been very well described by Stores (1986), who has distinguished between different types. Some children appear almost 'zombie-like', are unable to speak and may even be unable to walk. Others may simply appear a little quieter than usual. The present author has examined a number of these children on split-screen video–EEG recordings, confirming the findings of previous authors that there is no direct relationship between the amount of EEG abnormality and the clinical state of the child. Some children are very impaired with only moderately frequent discharges whilst others are able to function remarkably well despite almost continuous spike and wave on the EEG. The importance of suspecting the condition cannot be overemphasized. It is easy to diagnose with an EEG recording, and intravenous medication will often, although not always, quickly bring the child out of the severely impaired state.

Sleep disturbance

Although most clinicians specializing in epilepsy are well aware that some children have silent nocturnal seizures that affect their school performance the following day, perhaps insufficient attention has been given to the quality of the sleep itself. Children who are tired in the classroom are unlikely to be receptive to educational input (Stores, 1990).

Treatment of the epilepsy

Effects of antiepileptic medication

Drugs can affect learning and behaviour in both beneficial and deleterious ways. Phenobarbitone, primidone and benzodiazepines are particularly notorious for their adverse effects on childhood behaviour. One of the surprising findings of the Holdsworth and Whitmore (1974a) study was that phenobarbitone seemed to be associated with better performance in the children they studied. This suggests that, in some children at least, the benefits of seizure control outweigh any adverse effects of this drug. Unfortunately this is not always the case. A particularly interesting series of investigations has been carried out by Thompson, Trimble and co-workers (Thompson and Trimble, 1982; Trimble and Thompson, 1985; Trimble, 1990). Additional studies of note are those of Andrewes et al (1986), Gallassi et al (1988), Trimble (1988), and Richens (1989).

The consensus of opinion is that phenytoin seems to impair cognitive function and educational progress. Carbamazepine and valproate do not seem to have this effect. However, there is a suggestion that it might be wise to avoid higher levels of these drugs. Drug combinations are also to be avoided; monotherapy is preferred.

The relatively new drugs, vigabatrin and lamotrigine, are worthy of particular comment in this context. Vigabatrin can occasionally precipitate psychosis in adults and teenagers. It can also be associated with gross behavioural disturbance in some children. It is nevertheless a useful drug, particularly in treating partial seizures.

Lamotrigine is remarkable in making many patients, both adults and children, feel better. The carefully conducted study by Smith et al (1992), using a double-blind design, has shown that patients were significantly better on scales of mastery and on one of the mood scales. The reasons for these results remain unclear. However, Besag (1992) has shown that lamotrigine is very effective in suppressing spike-and-wave discharges. In half the children treated, frequent spike-and-wave discharges resistant to other antiepileptic medication were reduced by more than 80%. Not surprisingly, the children appeared alert, happy and more in control of their lives. D. Smith and D. Chadwick (personal communication) have argued that a similar explanation could not apply to the adults they studied, who had a very different form of epilepsy, with no evidence of frequent abnormal EEG discharges between the obvious seizures. It is of particular interest to note that lamotrigine may be effective in a significant proportion of people with the Lennox–Gastaut syndrome, both adults and children, as reported by Oller et al (1991). Gibbs and colleagues (1992) also reported better educational progress in a small series of children taking lamotrigine, some of whom had learning disability.

In summary, carbamazepine and sodium valproate remain the first-line antiepileptic drugs. Phenobarbitone, primidone, phenytoin and the benzo-diazepines should be avoided in children, as they may all affect educational progress. The roles of vigabatrin and lamotrigine need to be elucidated further, but it seems that lamotrigine may be associated with an improvement in educational progress in at least some children.

Effects of epilepsy neurosurgery

The commonest epilepsy neurosurgical operation carried out is temporal lobectomy. After this operation, function may be diminished, increased or remain the same. In general, major deficits do not result. Since a large proportion of the subjects will be rendered seizure-free, with obvious benefits to educational continuity, the balance is weighted in favour of proceeding with neurosurgery in appropriately selected cases.

Hemispherectomy carried out for children who have an early, major unilateral brain insult, including those with Rasmussen's syndrome (progressive hemi-atrophy of the brain), can have a very favourable outcome with major improvements both in seizure control and behaviour (for a review see Goodman, 1986).

Reactions to the epilepsy

Pazzaglia and Frank-Pazzaglia (1976) commented on the high proportion of teachers who felt poorly prepared for having children with epilepsy in their class. Reactions of other pupils and their parents were also very unfavourable if the child had seizures at school (see above). Over-protection and rejection can be very damaging to the child, both in terms of personal and educational progress. Another factor, which is less often discussed, is teasing by other children. If the child is the only individual in the school with epilepsy, he or she may be subjected to merciless teasing. It was clear from the Pazzaglia and Frank-Pazzaglia study that closer co-operation between teachers, psychologists and physicians was very much desired. Education, not only of professionals but also of the parents of other pupils and of the pupils themselves, could do much to reduce the morbidity of epilepsy in school.

Associated brain damage

Most children with epilepsy do not have brain damage, but epilepsy may either be caused by brain damage or rarely may cause it, e.g. through prolonged status epilepticus. These concepts are discussed further below. The importance of carrying out careful psychometric assessments to determine the educational strengths and weaknesses of the child presenting with educational difficulty cannot be overemphasized. There has been a recent unfortunate tendency to avoid carrying out such assessments. In the absence of the information, it is difficult to plan appropriate interventions.

Causes that are equally applicable to those without epilepsy

Educational difficulties can have a large number of causes, and the child with epilepsy is subject to all the usual ones. The fact that he or she is having educational difficulties does not necessarily mean the epilepsy is to blame. If other reasons are sought, they can be corrected.

EPILEPSY AND MENTAL HANDICAP

There are some obvious situations in which epilepsy and mental handicap can occur together. A child who has gross brain damage from any cause is much more liable to have seizures. In this case, the brain damage has caused both the intellectual impairment and the epilepsy. In a minority of children, prolonged status epilepticus can cause clear-cut brain damage. The most interesting situation is, however, when the apparent brain damage appears to be insidious in onset.

Epilepsy and mental handicap has been reviewed by the present author (Besag, 1988a). The concept of deterioration in people with epilepsy is not new. The writings of Aretaeus the Cappadocian, AD 81–138 and, in the last century, William Gowers left little doubt about some type of association. It is important to highlight both aspects of what Gowers said in the two following statements: 'The mental state of epileptics, as is well-known, frequently presents deterioration . . . every grade of intellectual defect may be met with down to actual imbecility' and 'the mental state must not be regarded in all instances as entirely the effect of the disease. It is certainly, in some, the expression of cerebral imperfection of which the epilepsy is another manifestation. . .'. Reviews by Brown and Reynolds (1981), Addy (1987) and Lesser et al (1986) contain much helpful material. Rodin has also been interested in this field over a number of years, and has published valuable material (Rodin, 1968; Rodin et al, 1986).

It was suggested in a previous review by the present author (Besag, 1988a) that the confusion and conflicting answers embodied in the large amount of literature that has been published on this subject might usefully be examined by asking a number of questions:

1.   Is epilepsy associated with deterioration?
2.   Does epilepsy cause deterioration?

3.   Does deterioration cause epilepsy?
4.   Do both epilepsy and deterioration reflect some underlying causative brain abnormality?
5.   When epilepsy and cognitive deterioration occur together, what factors might be important?

The main points are summarized, and reference should be made to the previous paper (Besag, 1988c) for a more detailed review.

Is epilepsy associated with deterioration?

A series of studies carried out at Lingfield, commencing in 1924 with the report of 14 tests on 150 students at this residential special centre for children with epilepsy, have shown that a falling IQ can occur in some cases. Tylor Fox (1924) found that 8% of the children deteriorated by more than ten points in successive Binet tests. Cookson (1927) found 'marked mental deficiency' in 26 of 100 children examined. Dawson and Conn (1929) found that 16 of 21 children deteriorated by more than ten IQ points. Chaudhry and Pond (1961) compared a group of 28 children with epilepsy who deteriorated and a control group of 28 who did not. Hung (1968) studied 500 adults and children with epilepsy; approximately one quarter were intellectually impaired. The studies of Pond and Bidwell (1960), Rutter et al (1970), Pazzaglia and Frank-Pazzaglia (1976), Stores and Hart (1976), Seidenberg et al (1986) and Corbett et al (1975) all appeared to confirm that a proportion of children with epilepsy have a falling IQ. However, later studies by the Lingfield group, e.g. Besag (1988c) showed that most of the children with a falling IQ did not have a falling mental age. The Lingfield studies contain the largest reported group of closely examined children with a falling IQ. Corbett and colleagues (Corbett, 1985; Corbett et al, 1985a,b) found that 50% of 160 students with epilepsy at St Piers Lingfield had an IQ reduction of more than 15 points and that 16% fell by more than 30 points in sequential tests. Examination of initial IQ, age, sex, age of seizure onset, seizure frequency, EEG abnormality and antiepileptic drugs showed no significant association with the fall in IQ. In an ongoing study by Besag (1988c) only two of the children with falling IQ were found to have a falling mental age. In one of these, who was subject to frequent bouts of non-convulsive status epilepticus, the mental age was found not to have fallen permanently. It appears that these children do not deteriorate in *absolute* terms: the mental age does not rise as quickly as the chronological age, resulting in a falling IQ.

Does epilepsy cause deterioration?

There is no doubt that epilepsy can cause deterioration in children who have prolonged bouts of status epilepticus. There is also the possibility that serious injury in seizures, or possibly even repeated less-serious head injury, might cause damage. However, in most children with epilepsy who have a falling IQ there is no obvious explanation. The definition of what is meant by 'deterioration' requires some clarification. It is interesting to consider that, although a child with a slowly rising mental age is not deteriorating in terms of losing skills, because the IQ is falling, they may change slowly from being of 'normal' intelligence to falling within the range of mental handicap. In terms of social and educational status this certainly represents a deterioration, although the child has lost no skills. Paediatricians like to see the development of a child following an appropriate centile on a chart. When it fails to keep pace, this is viewed with alarm. How these concepts should apply in the current context is difficult to decide. This is not only a semantic problem but also an educational, social and philosophical one.

Does deterioration cause epilepsy?

As stated in the introductory comments of this section, it is quite clear that trauma can cause brain damage and that the brain damage in turn can result in epilepsy. Meningitis and neurodegenerative diseases, particularly those affecting the grey matter, can also cause seizures; examples are Alzheimer's disease, subacute sclerosing panencephalitis and Batten's disease. A suggestion that has been made from time to time involves a much less obvious mechanism. Rodin (see Rodin et al, 1986) has been one of the workers who raised the question of the possibility of a subgroup of children with epilepsy who have some unknown cerebral disturbance predisposing to seizures and persisting to 'reassert itself in later life', leading to cerebral degeneration. This would explain the finding that some subjects whose seizures are controlled and who are either on or off antiepileptic medication, still appear to have some underlying mechanism causing deterioration or preventing appropriate intellectual development. A similar concept was suggested by Besag (1988c).

When epilepsy and cognitive impairment occur together, which factors might be important?

Earlier work suggested that intellectual deterioration occurred only in those cases where there was obvious pre-existing organic brain damage (e.g. Lennox, 1942; Yacorzynski and Arieff, 1942). However, subsequent work, including that of the Lingfield group, has shown this is not necessarily the case. Later studies have also, in general, failed to demonstrate any clear effect of age of seizure onset, duration of epilepsy, seizure type, seizure frequency or antiepileptic drugs. With regard to the last of these factors, phenytoin has been associated with educational and intellectual problems to the extent that Corbett et al (1985a) proposed a chronic phenytoin encephalopathy. However, this drug is now used so seldom to treat childhood epilepsy in developed countries that the effect has been difficult to confirm in later studies. Amongst the more recent and important epidemiological studies, Ellenberg et al (1985) concluded that epilepsy caused no significant deterioration in the group they studied (see also above) when sibling controls were used. However, as has been pointed out by Besag (1988c), epidemiological studies of large groups may fail to identify an important subgroup of children who have a falling IQ. Selected populations are not representative, but the study of them is very important in establishing that, for a subgroup of children with epilepsy, failure to develop at the appropriate rate, with the resulting fall in IQ, definitely does occur.

State-dependent and permanent intellectual impairment

It is very important to distinguish between these two situations. The commonest cause of state-dependent intellectual impairment in the population as a whole is alcohol intoxication. This example is given because it is so familiar to the general public. The analogy to children who have toxic levels of antiepileptic drugs is all too obvious and unfortunately not uncommon. However, another important cause of state-dependent intellectual impairment relates to the seizures themselves. Non-convulsive status epilepticus has already been discussed in this chapter. Assessments of intellectual function carried out while a child is in this state may lead to the incorrect conclusion that irreversible damage has occurred. It is interesting to note, although difficult to prove, that paediatricians who have considerable experience of children with frequent prolonged bouts of non-convulsive status epilepticus suspect that the state-dependent intellectual impairment caused by this condition may, if it continues for long enough, also produce a degree of permanent impairment. The other situation in which state-dependent impairment may occur is in the postictal phase. In children who have occasional seizures this will be obvious, and allowance can be made for it. However, if a child has four or five seizures a day, he or she may never have the opportunity to recover fully before the next seizure occurs. This potentially treatable situation mimics permanent intellectual impairment. If better antiepileptic control can be achieved, the child may emerge from the state-dependent postictal impairment, proving that it was not permanent. Children who are treated with antiepileptic drugs that cause gross behavioural disturbance (see above) may also show state-dependent impairment on testing.

From these comments it is clear that state-dependent impairment may be ictal, postictal or the result of drug effects. State-dependent and permanent impairment may occur together. In some cases, state-dependent impairment may even cause permanent impairment. Because state-dependent impairment is potentially reversible it is of the utmost importance to seek it energetically and to manage the child appropriately, to try to reverse the effect, allowing full use of whatever intellect he or she may have.

O'Donohoe (1994) has decried the term 'childhood epilepsy' on the basis that this is a group of conditions that vary from the benign to the very serious. It is for this reason that he has entitled his book *Epilepsies of Childhood* (not epilepsy of childhood). For example, the prognosis of West's syndrome on one hand and that of benign focal seizures on the other is very different indeed. However, even children who do not have one of the syndromes with a bad prognosis may show a falling IQ.

With regard to the association between mental handicap and epilepsy, the following conclusions may be drawn. Brain damage may cause both mental handicap and epilepsy. Several studies have shown that children with mental handicap are much more likely to have epilepsy. Because of this, cross-sectional studies of children with epilepsy will show an increased number with mental handicap. This does not, of course, imply that the epilepsy causes the mental handicap. Epidemiological studies of large groups have failed to establish definite deterioration in children with epilepsy. However, sequential testing on selected groups has shown a falling IQ in a subgroup. The reasons for this failure to develop at the expected rate remain unclear. In most cases the children do not deteriorate in absolute terms: the mental age does not fall; instead it rises slowly or, at worst, remains stationary. This concept has major implications because the parent of a child with a falling IQ may think that this represents inexorable loss of skills, when this is not the case. Status epilepticus can undoubtedly cause brain damage and should be treated promptly. There is a possibility that very prolonged non-convulsive status epilepticus might also cause some permanent damage. It is very important to distinguish between state-dependent, and potentially reversible intellectual impairment and permanent intellectual impairment; the former should always be treated energetically. Whenever a child actually loses skills there is usually an identifiable cause that must be sought carefully. Some epilepsy syndromes, for example West's syndrome and the Lennox–Gastaut syndrome, seem much more likely to be associated with poor intellectual outcome. The literature remains conflicting in terms of causes of IQ fall in children with epilepsy. Although the results fail to reach significance in most of the studies, there is a suggestion that early age of onset, frequent seizures, prolonged seizures, association with pre-existing brain damage and mixed seizure type may all contribute.

DIAGNOSIS, ASSESSMENT, INVESTIGATION AND MANAGEMENT OF THE CHILD WITH EPILEPSY AND EDUCATIONAL DIFFICULTY

The most important factor in diagnosing, assessing and managing the child with epilepsy and educational difficulty is taking a meticulous history. This does *not* simply mean reviewing past notes, although this is an essential part of the assessment. Re-taking the history from the parents and other key informants may clarify the situation to such an extent that intervention becomes possible in a child for whom all options had apparently already been tried. The first step is to take a detailed history of the evolution of the child's development and the epilepsy; this must include a history of schooling. Neurological examination of the child should be carried out, as well as psychometric testing. When this information is taken together, it may be possible to place the problem into one or more of the categories listed above. Appropriate, rational intervention can then be planned.

Most epilepsy specialists will be able to recount the histories of children who were considered to be 'hopeless cases' and who, after reassessment and appropriate management, improved markedly. Two brief examples might suffice here.

Patient 1. A 19-year-old woman was having up to 11 complex partial seizures a day. She had been seen by many specialists in the past. A careful history was taken. Her past notes comprised four volumes. It took 10 hours to summarize these records. It emerged that she had been treated with all the appropriate antiepileptic drugs and had been referred for neurosurgery but was unsuitable. However, one of the antiepileptic drugs had not been used for about 5 years. This was recommenced and she became seizure-free and remained so during the ensuing follow-up period of 18 months. Her whole persona changed from being someone who sat hunched in her chair, lacking any self-confidence, to that of a personable young woman who walked around with her head held high. The hours taken gathering the information had been time well spent.

Patient 2. This 16-year-old lad had a single seizure at 5 years of age and subsequent recurrent seizures from 7 years. He then had 20 to 30 bouts of status epilepticus, lasting at least 20 min. He developed mixed epilepsy, including atonic drop attacks. Computed tomography (CT) showed a mild degree of cerebral atrophy. The boy sat rocking in his chair, disoriented in time and space, being unable to string words together into a sentence. His mental state was reminiscent of that of an elderly person with dementia. He wandered at night, not knowing where he was. The introduction of a second-line antiepileptic drug, which had not previously been tried, transformed him. His seizures were completely controlled and he began reading again. He was able to carry out sensible conversations, to take an active part in domestic chores and to socialize with his peers. This was a dramatic case of state-dependent postictal intellectual impairment in someone who was having such frequent seizures that he did not have time to recover from one seizure before the next occurred. He may also have been having some subtle seizure activity, impairing his performance. When the state-dependent component of the intellectual impairment was reversed, the patient was able to function at a level that delighted his parents and carers, who had previously thought that his course would be one of relentless deterioration.

The following scheme might be adopted for the diagnosis, assessment, investigation and management of epilepsy in a child who is experiencing educational difficulty. The scheme would need to be tailored to the individual child.

1. Re-take a meticulous history, including accounts from people who have known the child for a long period, preferably the parents, documenting development and seizure history, in particular.
2. Examine the child, particularly seeking possible diagnoses that might affect prognosis or genetic counselling advice, for example the stigmata of tuberose sclerosis.
3. Review past records carefully.
4. Carry out basic blood tests, including full blood count, biochemistry and antiepileptic blood level determinations to establish compliance and evaluate possible toxicity. Consider special investigations, e.g.

blood amino acids or urine organic acids, if a metabolic disorder is suspected.

5. Carry out appropriate EEG investigations including, where applicable, overbreathing when absence seizures are suspected, a sleep EEG when complex partial seizures are suspected, overnight EEG monitoring when silent nocturnal seizures or sleep disturbance may be occurring, and prolonged monitoring for frequent subtle seizures, which do not always appear on routine EEG.

6. Neuroimaging with CT and, if possible, magnetic resonance imaging. To identify mesial temporal sclerosis, which may be suitable for neurosurgery, and migrational defects, as well as other brain pathology that might be remediable.

7. Carry out psychometric testing to determine where strengths and weaknesses lie, before designing a suitable educational programme.

8. Explain to the child and the family any epilepsy-related phenomena that might have been described, for example aura or automatisms, emphasizing that epilepsy is a common condition in childhood and reassuring the family that there are many other children who exhibit these epilepsy-related phenomena.

9. Consider a re-trial of any first-line drugs that have not been used in the past 4 years. Consider second-line drugs.

10. Seek a neurosurgical opinion for localization-related seizures that might be amenable to focal resection and for children who have had an early insult to one hemisphere, who might be suitable for hemispherectomy.

11. Examine the interaction between the epilepsy and educational failure against the criteria listed in the section on educational failure.

12. Support and counsel the child and family.

13. Provide information and support to teaching staff.

14. If the child is not coping in a mainstream or local special school, consider a period of assessment and treatment at an epilepsy special school.

THE ROLE OF SPECIAL SCHOOLS FOR CHILDREN WITH EPILEPSY

Most children with epilepsy achieve good seizure control and do not require special schooling (for a review see Besag 1986, 1988a,b, this section is based on English educational provision, comparable facilities and legislation apply in other developed countries). Some require additional input in a mainstream school or may need to be educated in a local special school. An important minority have special needs that may be very demanding on teachers, parents, medical services and other professionals. They may require very specialized services that are not available in the local area. If efficient use is to be made of the necessarily limited local services, a proportion of this small number of children who make large demands on the services should be educated in specialist establishments capable of meeting

Table 2. Reasons for referral.

Difficult epilepsy
  Frequent seizures
  Injury in seizures
  Risk of status epilepticus
  Variable seizure frequency
  Postictal problems
  Antiepileptic drug problems
  Inadequate control
  Difficult-to-recognize epilepsy
Other medical problems
Cognitive problems
Behavioural problems
Peer group problems
Family and social problems
Psychiatric problems
Multiple problems

their needs. These comments are entirely consistent with the much mis-quoted English Warnock Report 1978 and the Education Act 1981 which followed it. The Warnock Report emphasized that there would be a continuing need for special residential schools for a minority of children whose overall educational needs could not reasonably be met in any other way. Table 2 lists the reasons for referral and provides an explanation of the term 'difficult epilepsy'. A more detailed discussion of each of these categories can be found in a previous review (Besag, 1986). The reasons why these factors might interfere with the educational progress of the child have largely been discussed in the foregoing sections of this chapter.

The emphasis within the special school is on close teamwork. Medical staff with specialist teachers, care workers, psychologists, physiotherapists, occupational therapists, speech therapists and nursing staff offer a comprehensive assessment of the needs of the whole child. The skills of the professionals are combined to fulfil these needs. Some children are referred for brief assessments, covering two school terms. Requests are occasionally received for shorter periods of assessment. In my opinion, it is inadvisable to offer very brief assessments of children with epilepsy who have complex problems and who have not been managed satisfactorily on an outpatient basis. Changes in epilepsy generally take place slowly. Quick decisions may be incorrectly based, since epilepsy tends to fluctuate. The purpose of the assessment lasting two school terms is to determine the special needs of the child, to begin interventions to fulfil these needs, to document meticulously the up-to-date situation towards the end of the assessment period and to meet with all those concerned, including the parents together with professionals both in the school and from the local education authority, to formulate a plan aimed at fulfilling the future needs of the child. The conclusion may be that the child can return to the local area or it may be that a longer period at the specialist school is the best way, for the moment, of fulfilling his or her needs.

The Warnock Report (1978), in agreement with an earlier report, stated that special schools offer a form of positive discrimination for children whose needs cannot adequately be met with local provision. The needs of most children with epilepsy can be met satisfactorily by the local services but it is very important for the parents and professionals concerned to recognize when this is not the case and to refer the child to the epilepsy special school, rather than to allow a deteriorating situation that may be difficult to reverse, with lost educational opportunities, inadequate assessment facilities and consequent lack of appropriate medical intervention. Early referral for assessment and treatment to an epilepsy special school in some cases is a good way of preventing the escalating problems. The needs of the child must come first.

CONCLUSION

The epilepsies of childhood cover a wide variety of situations from the benign to the serious. In addition, there are many individual factors in each case that need careful assessment. It is important for professionals to be realistic in their approach to the education of the child with epilepsy. Although many children encounter no significant educational problems, quite a high proportion will require some help. A minority will require intensive help, which should not be delayed. Meticulous assessment enables the causes of educational difficulty to be determined and rational intervention to be arranged.

SUMMARY

Epidemiological studies have consistently shown that up to one half of children with epilepsy will encounter some educational difficulty. Some of the possible reasons for the difficulty are classified in this chapter and form a framework against which rational management of the child can be undertaken. The educational difficulty may be the consequence of organic factors, either related or unrelated to the epilepsy, but environmental factors arising from unfavourable responses to the epilepsy may also be important.

Epilepsy may rarely result from or cause brain damage, in turn causing learning disability. In some instances the damage is preventable, for example that resulting from prolonged seizures.

A small subgroup of children with epilepsy have a falling IQ but they do not usually lose skills in absolute terms unless there is some identifiable cause such as a neurodegenerative disease or status epilepticus. Any child who does appear to be losing skills should be investigated energetically because a cause can usually be found and may need specific treatment. The importance of distinguishing state-dependent, potentially reversible impairment from permanent impairment cannot be overemphasized.

Most children with epilepsy should be educated in a mainstream school, but some will require additional help or alternative schooling. A small proportion have needs that cannot reasonably be met with local facilities, and they may require the diagnostic or management resources of an epilepsy special school.

REFERENCES

Addy D (1987) Cognitive function in children with epilepsy. *Developmental Medicine and Child Neurology* **29:** 394–404.

Andrewes DG, Bullen JG, Tomlinson L et al (1986) A comparative study of the cognitive effects of phenytoin and carbamazepine in new referrals with epilepsy. *Epilepsia* **27:** 128–134.

Besag FMC (1986) The role of the special centres for children with epilepsy. In Oxley J & Stores G (eds) *Symposium on Epilepsy and Education, Royal College of Physicians*, pp 65–71. Manchester: Medical Tribune Group.

Besag FMC (1988a) Schooling the child with epilepsy. *The Royal College of General Practitioners Members' Reference Book*, pp 370–372. London: RCGP.

Besag FMC (1988b) Which school for the child with epilepsy? *MED* **2(2):** 16–17.

Besag FMC (1988c) Cognitive deterioration in children with epilepsy. In Trimble MR & Reynolds EH (eds) *Symposium on Epilepsy, Behaviour and Cognitive Function, Stratford upon Avon, 1987*, pp 113–127. Chichester: John Wiley.

Besag FMC (1992) Lamotrigine: paediatric experience. In Richens A (ed.) *Clinical Update on Lamotrigine: A Novel Antiepileptic Agent*, pp 53–60. Tunbridge Wells: Wells Medical.

Besag FMC (1993) Epilepsy, learning and behaviour: an overview. *Journal of Educational and Child Psychology* **10(1):** 36–45.

Besag FMC, Corbett JA, Fowler M & Pool F (1989a) Cognitive deterioration in children with epilepsy at a residential special school. *Abstracts of 18th International Epilepsy Congress* **174:** 44.

Besag FMC, Loney G, Waudby E et al (1989b) A multidisciplinary approach to epilepsy, learning difficulties and behavioural problems. *Journal of Educational and Child Psychology* **6(2):** 18–24.

Binnie CD (1980) Detection of transitory cognitive impairment during epileptiform EEG discharges: problems in clinical practice. In Kulig BM, Meinardi H & Stores G (eds) *Epilepsy and Behaviour*, pp 91–97. Lisse: Swets and Zeitlinger.

Brown SW & Reynolds EH (1981) Cognitive impairment in epileptic patients. In Reynolds EH & Trimble M (eds) *Epilepsy and Psychiatry*, pp 147–164. Edinburgh: Churchill Livingstone.

Chaudhry MR & Pond DA (1961) Mental deterioration in epileptic children. *Journal of Neurology, Neurosurgery and Psychiatry* **24:** 213–219.

Cookson SH (1927) An analysis of 100 cases of fits in children. *Archives of Disease in Childhood* **II:** 178.

Corbett JA (1985) Epilepsy as part of a handicapping condition. In Ross E & Reynolds E (eds) *Paediatric Perspectives on Epilepsy*, pp 79–89. Chichester: John Wiley.

Corbett JA, Harris R & Robinson R (1975) Epilepsy. In Wortis J (ed.) *Mental Retardation and Developmental Disabilities*, vol. VII, pp 79–111. New York: Bruner Mazel.

Corbett JA, Trimble M & Nicol TC (1985a) Behavioural and cognitive impairments in children with epilepsy: the long-term effects of anticonvulsant therapy. *Journal of the American Academy of Child Psychiatry* **24:** 17–23.

Corbett JA, Besag FMC, James A & White S (1985b) *Cognitive and behavioural impairment in children with epilepsy. Lingfield study II—preliminary analysis*. Presented to the British Paediatric Neurology Association, Sheffield, January 1985.

Dawson S & Conn JCM (1929) The intelligence of epileptic children. *Archives of Disease in Childhood* **4:** 142–151.

Ellenberg JH, Hirtz DG & Nelson KB (1985) Do seizures in children cause intellectual deterioration? *Annals of Neurology* **18:** 389.

Fenton GW (1972) Epilepsy and automatism. *British Journal of Hospital Medicine* **7:** 57–64.

Gallassi R, Morreale A, Lorusso S et al (1988) Epilepsy presenting as memory disturbances. *Epilepsia* **29(5):** 624–629.

Gibbs J, Appleton RE, Rosenbloom L & Yeun WC (1992) Lamotrigine for intractable childhood epilepsy: a preliminary communication. *Developmental Medicine and Child Neurology* **34:** 369–371.

Goodman R (1986) Hemispherectomy and its alternatives in the treatment of intractable epilepsy in patients with infantile hemiplegia. *Developmental Medicine and Child Neurology* **28:** 251–258.

Green JB & Hartlage LC (1971) Comparative performance of epileptic and non-epileptic children and adolescents. *Diseases of the Nervous System* **32**: 418–421.

Holdsworth L & Whitmore K (1974a) A study of children with epilepsy attending ordinary schools. I: Their seizure patterns, progress and behaviour in school. *Developmental Medicine and Child Neurology* **16**: 746–758.

Holdsworth L & Whitmore K (1974b) A study of children with epilepsy attending ordinary schools. II: Information and attitudes held by their teachers. *Developmental Medicine and Child Neurology* **16**: 759–765.

Hung T-P (1968) Intellectual impairment and behaviour disorder in 500 epileptic patients. *Proceedings of the Australian Association of Neurology* **5**: 163–170.

Knox SJ (1968) Epileptic automatism and violence. *Medical Science and Law* **8**: 96.

Kurtz Z, Tookey P & Ross E (1987) The epidemiology of epilepsy in childhood. In Ross E, Chadwick D & Crawford R (eds) *Epilepsy in Young People*, pp 13–21. Chichester: John Wiley.

Lennox WG (1942) Brain injury drugs and environment as causes of mental decay in epileptics. *American Journal of Psychiatry* **99**: 174–180.

Lesser RP, Luders H, Wyllie E et al (1986) Mental deterioration in epilepsy. *Epilepsia* **27 (supplement 2)**: S105–S123.

Lishman WA (ed.) (1978) *Organic Psychiatry*, 320 pp. London: Blackwell.

Marston D, Binnie C & Besag FMC (1993) Effects of transitory cognitive impairment on psychosocial functioning of children with epilepsy: a therapeutic trial. *Developmental Medicine and Child Neurology* **35**: 574–581.

O'Donohoe NV (1994) *Epilepsies of Childhood*, 2nd edn. London: Butterworth-Heinemann.

Oller L, Russi A & Oller Daurella L (1991) Lamotrigine in Lennox–Gastaut syndrome. *Epilepsia* **32 (supplement 1)**: 58.

Ounsted C, Lindsay J & Norman R (1966) Biological factors in temporal lobe epilepsy. *Clinics in Developmental Medicine*, no. 22. London: Spastics Society–Heinemann Medical.

Pazzaglia P & Frank-Pazzaglia L (1976) Record in grade school of pupils with epilepsy: an epidemiological study. *Epilepsia* **17**: 361–366.

Pond DA & Bidwell BH (1960) A survey of epilepsy in fourteen general practices. II: Social and psychological aspects. *Epilepsia* **1**: 285–299.

Richens A (1989) *Educational and Child Psychology* **6(2)**: 44–49.

Rodin EA (1968) In Thomas C (ed.) *The Prognosis of Patients with Epilepsy*. Illinois: Springfield.

Rodin EA, Schmaltz S & Twitty G (1986) Intellectual functions of patients with childhood-onset epilepsy. *Developmental Medicine and Child Neurology* **28**: 25–33.

Ross EM, Peckham CS, West PB & Butler NR (1980) Epilepsy in childhood: findings from the National Child Development Study. *British Medical Journal* **1**: 207–210.

Rutter M, Graham P & Yule W (1970) A neuropsychiatric study in childhood. *Clinics in Developmental Medicine*, nos 35–36 SIMP. London: Heinemann Medical.

Seidenberg M, Beck N, Geisser M et al (1986) Academic achievement of children with epilepsy. *Epilepsia* **27**: 753–759.

Sillanpää M (1983) Social functioning and seizure status of young adults with onset of epilepsy in childhood. An epidemiological 20-year follow-up study. *Acta Neurologica Scandinavica* **68 (supplement 96)**: 1–81.

Sillanpää M (1990) Prognosis of children with epilepsy. In Sillanpää M, Johannessen SI, Blennow G & Dam M (eds) *Paediatric Epilepsy*, pp 341–368. Petersfield: Wrightson Biomedical.

Sillanpää M (1992) Epilepsy in children: prevalence, disability and handicap. *Epilepsia* **33(3)**: 444–449.

Smith D, Chadwick D, Baker G et al (1992) Quality of life and reduction in seizure severity produced by lamotrigine. In Richens A (ed.) *Clinical Update on Lamotrigine: A Novel Antiepileptic Agent*, pp 43–52. Tunbridge Wells: Wells Medical.

Stores G (1971) Cognitive function in children with epilepsy. *Developmental Medicine and Child Neurology* **13**: 390–393.

Stores G (1973) Studies of attention and seizure disorders. *Developmental Medicine and Child Neurology* **15**: 376–382.

Stores G (1975) Behavioural effects of anti-epileptic drugs. *Developmental Medicine and Child Neurology* **17**: 647–658.

Stores G (1977) Behaviour disturbance and type of epilepsy in children attending ordinary school. In Penry JK (ed.) *Epilepsy: Proceedings of the Eighth International Symposium*, pp 245–249. New York: Raven Press.

Stores G (1978) School-children with epilepsy at risk for learning and behaviour problems. *Developmental Medicine and Child Neurology* **20:** 502–508.

Stores G (1981) Problems of learning and behaviour in children with epilepsy. In Reynolds EH & Trimble ER (eds) *Epilepsy and Psychiatry*, pp 33–48. London: Churchill Livingstone.

Stores G (1986) Psychological aspects of non-convulsive status epilepticus in children. *Journal of Child Psychology and Psychiatry* **27:** 575–582.

Stores G (1989) Epilepsy and the schoolchild. *Educational and Child Psychology* **6(2):** 8–10.

Stores G (1990) Electroencephalographic parameters in assessing the cognitive function of children with epilepsy. *Epilepsia* **31 (supplement 4):** S45–49.

Stores G & Hart J (1976) Reading skills of children with generalized or focal epilepsy attending ordinary school. *Developmental Medicine and Child Neurology* **18:** 705–716.

Stores G, Hart JA & Piran N (1978) Inattentiveness in school children with epilepsy. *Epilepsia* **19:** 169–175.

Thompson PJ & Trimble MR (1982) Comparative effects of anticonvulsant drugs on cognitive functioning. *British Journal of Clinical Practice* **18 (supplement):** 154–156.

Thompson PJ & Trimble MR (1983) Anticonvulsant drugs, cognitive function, and behaviour. *Epilepsia* **24 (supplement 1):** 555–563.

Trimble MR (1988) Anticonvulsant drugs: mood and cognitive function. In Trimble MR & Reynolds EH (eds) *Epilepsy, Behaviour and Cognitive Function*, pp 135–144. Chichester: John Wiley.

Trimble MR (1990) Antiepileptic drugs, cognitive function and behaviour in children: evidence from recent studies. *Epilepsia* **31 (supplement 4):** S30–S34.

Trimble MR & Thompson PJ (1985) Anticonvulsant drugs, cognitive function and behaviour. In Ross E & Reynolds E (eds) *Paediatric Perspectives on Epilepsy*, pp 141–148. Chichester: John Wiley.

Tylor Fox J (1924) The response of epileptic children to mental and educational tests. *British Journal of Medical Psychology* **4:** 235–238.

Verity CM & Ross EM (1985) Longitudinal studies of children's epilepsy. In Ross E & Reynolds E (eds) *Paediatric Perspectives on Epilepsy*, pp 133–140. Chichester: John Wiley.

Warnock Report (1978) *Special Educational Needs. Report of the Committee of Enquiry into the Education of Handicapped Children and Young People*. London: HMSO.

Yacorzynski GK & Arieff AJ (1942) Absence of deterioration in patients with non-organic epilepsy with especial reference to bromide therapy. *Journal of Nervous Mental Disorders* **95:** 687–697.

8

Neurophysiological investigation of epilepsy in children

COLIN D. BINNIE

As brain function depends on electrochemical processes, and epilepsy is a functional cerebral disorder, electrophysiological recording would appear to be a logical approach to the investigation of epilepsy. Indeed, electroencephalography (EEG) provides a non-invasive, inexpensive and repeatable means of assessing cerebral function of considerable practical clinical value in childhood epilepsy. However, EEG presents particular complexities in children because of the maturational changes that occur throughout childhood and adolescence. More generally, the areas of child neurology in which EEG is of most value are epilepsy as such and the various cerebral degenerative diseases, many of which give rise to seizures. It has a more questionable role as a 'soft' sign of cerebral dysfunction in general, and especially as evidence of epilepsy in children with obscure symptoms which may, or may not, be ictal in nature.

THE ELECTROENCEPHALOGRAM

Origin of the EEG

The EEG is a recording of cerebral electrical activity from the scalp. It is a spatiotemporal average of the activity of some 10^{10} cerebral neurones, and more specifically reflects that neuronal activity which is synchronous and produces electrical fields sufficiently widespread and suitably oriented to be detected from the scalp. In practice the EEG consists of the averaged synchronous postsynaptic potentials from radially oriented cortical neurones. Synchronous activity in such cells is mostly oscillatory in nature; consequently the ongoing activity of the EEG is rhythmic. Against this background, some brief transient EEG phenomena may occur, both normal and pathological, which owe their synchronicity to an intrinsic or external triggering event.

Synchronous, rhythmical neuronal activity arises in various ways. When not driven from external sources, both individual nerve cells and interconnected neuronal aggregates tend to display rhythmic discharge. There also exists anatomically discrete corticothalamic pacemakers and distributed

Baillière's Clinical Paediatrics—
Vol. 2, No. 3, August 1994
ISBN 0–7020–1862–7

systems of interacting neurones (for a review see Steriade et al, 1990). Rhythmic activity is modulated by afferent inputs. Thus it is suppressed during arousal by the activity of the ascending brain-stem reticular formation, which desynchronizes the EEG, increasing frequency and reducing amplitude. Conversely, deafferentation during sleep promotes synchrony, reflected in increased EEG amplitude and reduced frequency, and by an increased tendency for synchronous transients such as spikes to occur.

Recording the EEG

The EEG must be picked up by electrodes and amplified to drive a display device; traditionally this was a chart recorder, but increasingly visual display units are used. The EEG is of much lower amplitude than some other familiar bio-electric signals such as the ECG, of the order of 10–200 μV, and is consequently more difficult to record. Particular difficulties arise from artefacts, from biological sources such as the eyes (electro-oculogram) and scalp muscles (electromyogram), and from electrical interference due to electrode malfunction or environmental electrical fields. The problems can be largely overcome by meticulous technique, but this is particularly difficult to achieve in a child who may be distressed and unco-operative. Electrode preparation and application are crucial as low, stable, electrode potentials and contact resistances reduce susceptibility to physical interference. To minimize biological artefact it is necessary that the subject be still and relaxed, a state that is not easily obtained in infants and mentally handicapped or disturbed children.

Children's EEGs recorded in specialized paediatric centres are usually of far better technical quality than those obtained in less specialized departments, and technologists with special experience of children often succeed in obtaining good recordings without medication after others have failed even with heavy sedation. In the rare instances where it is really impossible to obtain an EEG without sedation or anaesthesia, one should consider whether the likely clinical value of the investigation justifies such measures. Preschool children will usually take a sedative antihistamine syrup, for instance trimeprazine 2 mg/kg, and older patients can be sedated with short-acting barbiturates, e.g. quinalbarbitone 100–150 mg. Before the last resort of general anaesthesia, which precludes a waking EEG, intramuscular droperidol may be tried.

Normal EEG phenomena in childhood and adolescence

As noted above, the EEG consists of a background of continuous *ongoing activity*, against which brief *transients* may occur. Ongoing EEG activities are divided by convention into four frequency bands: δ, below 4 cycles/s; θ, from 4 up to 8 cycles/s; α, from 8 up to 14 cycles/s; and β, from 14 cycles/s upwards. The EEG changes from birth, throughout childhood and adolescence, achieving a fairly stable adult pattern at about 22 years. This mature pattern will be described first, followed by the sequence of changes by which it is attained.

The mature EEG

Typically, the most prominent feature of the waking adult EEG is the α rhythm, an activity within the α frequency band, usually at about 9–10 cycles/s, with an amplitude of 50–100 μV appearing symmetrically at the back of the head. The α rhythm is of greatest amplitude in quiet wakefulness with closed eyes; it is reduced while the eyes are open and disappears in drowsiness and sleep. β Activity, of lower amplitude, usually some 10–20 μV, appears mainly over the frontocentral regions, typically at frequencies of about 18–25 cycles/s. θ Activity is present in variable amounts, generally with a bitemporal maximum, increasing in drowsiness. Particularly in young adults, θ activity of half the α frequency occurs posteriorly with a topography and response to eye-opening similar to that of the α rhythm ('slow α variant'). δ Activity is not generally visible in the mature waking EEG, although its presence can be demonstrated by computer analysis of the signals.

Drowsiness and sleep are characterized by marked EEG changes, which provide the basis of a widely used classification of sleep into five stages (Dement and Kleitman, 1957). In drowsiness (stage I) the α rhythm gives way to θ and/or β activity, and oculographic artefacts appear, indicating slow lateral eye movements. Transients consisting of isolated waves of sharp outline occur at the vertex in response to auditory stimuli ('vertex sharp transients'). In stage II, δ activity appears, β activity increases and spindled bursts of σ activity at about 14 cycles/s appear over the frontocentral regions. Arousal now produces a more complex waveform, typically the 'K complex': a sharp wave, a δ wave and a σ burst, maximal in the midline, generally at the vertex. Stages III and IV are characterized by increasing amounts of δ activity and a possible disappearance of σ in stage IV. After the first 90 min of sleep a new pattern appears, episodes of low amplitude activity accompanied by rapid lateral eye movements, which give this stage the name of REM sleep.

The neonatal EEG

The EEG of the full-term waking newborn consists mainly of diffuse δ activity. In sleep, two patterns occur: 'quiet sleep' is characterized by δ bursts interspersed with 6–10-s periods of relatively low amplitude ('tracé alternant'); in 'active sleep', which probably corresponds to REM in the mature EEG, δ activity is continuously present with superimposed faster components.

The first year

Over the first year the frequency of ongoing activity increases and a responsive posterior θ rhythm appears, which has a frequency of about 6 cycles/s by 12 months. From 3 to 12 months a Rolandic rhythm of 6–7 cycles/s is seen. From about 6 months the classical sleep stages are distinguishable. σ Activity appears at about 2 months and vertex sharp transients and K complexes at about 6 months.

During the preschool years, the α rhythm develops, increasing in frequency and responsiveness, to reach a frequency of 8–9 cycles/s by the age of 5 years. Underlying the α rhythm slower activities persist. The θ activity takes on the characteristics of a slow α variant and the δ becomes intermittent and focal over the posterior temporal regions. Through later childhood and adolescence, the slow α variant and posterior δ activity diminish, the posterior slow waves usually disappearing by 22 years, and the slow α variant a few years later. Drowsiness in early childhood is characterized by frontal θ activity, and slow activity in sleep shows a posterior maximum up to 3 years of age. Slow activity is present during REM sleep up to 5 years. Thereafter sleep patterns resemble those of adults.

Pathological EEG phenomena

A fundamental of EEG interpretation is that the EEG reflects cerebral function, and structural abnormality is manifest only in functional changes. Cerebral dysfunction produces a rather limited range of abnormal EEG phenomena, sometimes differing only quantitatively from normal findings, and usually of uncertain pathophysiology. It is often claimed that some 15% of normal children have abnormal EEGs, a proposition that implies at best a misunderstanding of normality, which is essentially a statistical concept. Findings that are common in health are normal, but rare variants found mainly in healthy subjects must also be regarded as normal.

Not only does the individual's EEG change with age and state of awareness, there is also considerable intersubject variance in normal children. Some EEG features are genetically determined. There are marked similarities between the records of monozygotic twins, both on visual assessment (Lennox et al, 1945) and using quantitative measures (Vogel, 1958; Dümermuth, 1968; Stassen et al, 1988). Various unusual or abnormal EEG features are also genetically determined (Doose and Gerken 1973).

Clinical EEG interpretation is subjective and depends on judgements that take into account the range of normal findings at different ages and in different states of awareness. The slower components become less with maturation and are increased in sleep and drowsiness. However, pathological slowing is a common feature of the abnormal EEG; thus it may be difficult to distinguish between the effects of immaturity, drowsiness and pathology.

Ongoing activities

Amplitude reduction. The most unequivocal EEG abnormality is a reduction in the amplitude of normal activity. This may reflect a lack of neuronal activity, due for instance to local or systemic anoxia, or a loss of neurones. Alternatively, amplitude reduction may be seen where conduction of signals from the cortex to the scalp is impaired, for instance by a subdural haematoma. Desynchronization of neuronal activity will also result in a reduction in amplitude; this is sometimes seen briefly at the onset of an epileptic seizure (an 'electrodecremental event').

Some normal children and adolescents constitutionally have low amplitude EEGs or show a marked voltage reduction when anxious. Amplitude reduction cannot usually be identified unless it is extreme, localized or asymmetrical, or transitory as in the case of an electro-decremental event. Asymmetry of normal activities greater than 50% is usually to be regarded as abnormal, reflecting disease on the side of lower amplitude.

Slowing. The amount of θ and δ activity is increased in many cerebral disorders, including cerebral hypoxia, oedema, raised intracranial pressure, inflammatory or degenerative processes, and intoxications. As these activities are normally present in a child's EEG, a minor excess may be identifiable only if also asymmetrical. In general, pathological slow frequency activity is most prominent over the region of greatest cerebral abnormality; however, this will not be the case if the underlying pathology also produces local amplitude reduction.

Excess β activity. The amplitude of β activity in children is very variable, and is increased in drowsiness and by various sedative drugs. Prominent β activity is rarely of clinical significance, but may sometimes raise the possibility that the patient is consuming non-prescribed drugs.

Altered responsiveness. A slowed α rhythm often shows a reduced response to eye opening or alerting, but α blocking shows considerable variation between healthy subjects and is also normally reduced in drowsiness. Again, it is the presence of asymmetry that often serves to confirm that poor responsiveness is pathological (there being less response on the more abnormal side).

Epileptiform activity

During an epileptic seizure the EEG typically shows spiky transients due to synchronous neuronal discharge. Waves of sharpened outline and less than 70 ms duration, standing out from ongoing activity, are called 'spikes', and those of 70–200 ms are 'sharp waves'. A spike is often followed by a slower wave to form a 'spike-and-wave' complex. These various spiky activities may occur in isolation or in bursts. During a seizure they typically show some form of progressive evolution of frequency (which generally slows) and of waveform, for instance from spikes to sharp waves to spike-and-wave activity.

These spiky phenomena also occur in the interictal state, between overt seizures, and are then more likely to be isolated or brief. They are also seen in some patients with cerebral disorders who do not apparently suffer from epilepsy. There is no universally agreed name for this class of EEG phenomena; the phrase 'epileptiform activity', which will be used here, acknowledges the association with epilepsy underlying the concept, whilst stressing that the term refers to the waveform and not to its possible clinical correlates.

Various sharp waveforms, unrelated to epilepsy, occur in normal subjects and have been a source of misunderstanding, and indeed of misdiagnosis. They are all recognizable by characteristic waveform, topography and circumstances of occurrence and should not be mistaken by a competent electroencephalographer for phenomena supporting a diagnosis of epilepsy. The most important of these normal spiky variants in paediatric practice are *six and 14 per second positive spikes* which occur in bursts at these two specific frequencies. They are positive at the site on the scalp where they are of greatest amplitude, a distinctive feature as most spikes are negative. Positive spikes occur in 20–30% of adolescents and young adults during drowsiness and light sleep. Their incidence may be marginally increased in various disorders, but their presence does not increase the likelihood that the subject has epilepsy.

Localized abnormalities

Amplitude reduction and slowing may be bilateral, asymmetrical or more localized. There may be a global reduction in the amplitude of all frequencies or only of fast activity. Local amplitude reduction generally reflects gross hypofunction or loss of underlying neurones.

Localized slowing also generally reflects underlying pathology, but is generated by the surviving dysfunctional neurones, not by an electrically inactive lesion such as a haematoma. Slowing therefore typically appears at the margins of a space-occupying lesion, whereas amplitude reduction may be seen over its centre.

Another important category of abnormal phenomena that may be localized is epileptiform activity; the significance of localized epileptiform discharges will be considered later.

Rhythms at a distance

Abnormal localized activities may appear over healthy cortex as a result of altered function of deep structures, so-called 'rhythms at a distance'.

FIRDA. Frontal intermittent rhythmic δ activity (FIRDA) appears in rhythmic bursts over the frontal regions, and is usually bilateral and synchronous. The frequency is 1.5–2.5 cycles/s, and the waveform either sinusoidal or saw-toothed. FIRDA occurs in a state of drowsiness or stupor; it is absent on full arousal and below stage I of sleep. It is seen in a variety of pathological conditions, but most commonly with diffuse disease involving grey and white matter (Gloor et al, 1968). It also occurs in metabolic and toxic disorders, status epilepticus and sometimes postictally, and with lesions of the diencephalon. It may thus, for instance, occur with thalamic tumours and with obstruction of the aqueduct.

Bitemporal θ activity. Temporal θ activity normally increases in drowsiness, but with pathological reduction of awareness excess bilateral rhythmic temporal or frontotemporal θ activity occurs, under circumstances similar to those producing FIRDA. It must be distinguished from the prominent frontal θ activity of drowsiness seen in preschool children.

Posterior slow waves. Posterior temporal slow waves are normal throughout childhood and adolescence. However, if they exceed the norm for the child's age, they may represent a non-specific abnormality after such cerebral insults as trauma, cerebrovascular accidents and severe hypoglycaemia. The slow waves may be more marked ipsilateral to a cerebral abnormality, but in general they share with normal maturational posterior temporal slow activity a tendency to predominate over the non-dominant hemisphere.

Sometimes there is evidence of brain-stem dysfunction in children with excess posterior slow activity, and in particular very slow occipital δ waves (of more than 1 s duration) are seen with posterior fossa lesions.

A characteristic rhythmic, usually bilateral, posterior slow activity at about 3 cycles/s occurs in some patients with childhood absence epilepsy. It may represent a variant of the spike-and-wave phenomenon (see below), as on overbreathing it often shows a gradual evolution of waveform and topography into typical generalized spike-and-wave discharges.

'Periodicity'

Some discontinuous abnormal EEG phenomena are regularly repetitive. A striking, but rare instance is the occurrence of stereotyped complexes of slow waves, spikes and sharp waves at 10–20-s intervals in subacute sclerosing panencephalitis. The conditions in which periodic phenomena appear are varied; they may have a common pathophysiology of diffuse dysfunction of both white and grey matter.

Other transients

Triphasic complexes comprise three slow waves of alternating polarity, which spread across the head from front to back with a small time lag. This is a sign of severe diffuse cerebral dysfunction, and is most often seen in metabolic disorders, notably hepatic encephalopathy.

Paroxysmal lateralized epileptiform discharges (PLEDs) are stereotyped sharp waves or sharp wave complexes occurring at intervals of about 1 s. They are generally widespread but lateralized to one hemisphere. PLEDs are found with localized structural disease, either acute or chronic, and possibly associated with more generalized cerebral dysfunction; examples include rapidly growing tumours, cerebrovascular accident, herpes simplex encephalitis, cerebral abscess and post-traumatic states.

Activation procedures

Various physiological stresses may be used to 'activate' the EEG with the aim of provoking clinically significant abnormalities; the chief of these are hyperventilation and photic stimulation.

Hyperventilation. This produces hypocapnoea, lowering systemic blood pressure, constricting the cerebral arterioles and thereby reducing blood flow in the brain. Most probably as a result of these changes in cerebral perfusion, overbreathing slows the EEG. The effects are most marked in the young, as indeed are the changes in end-tidal partial pressure of carbon dioxide. Children can be persuaded to overbreathe from about the age of 3 years, if necessary by means of play, for instance by blowing on a toy windmill. There is a general slowing of background activity, posterior slow waves increase and, if hyperventilation is performed effectively for 3 min, rhythmic bifrontal δ activity appears. Unfortunately, this response, which is entirely normal in the young, is sometimes misinterpreted as supporting a diagnosis of epilepsy. EEG abnormalities, including epileptiform activity may appear or increase on overbreathing. In particular generalized spike-and-wave discharges are likely to be activated, and any child with absence epilepsy can be relied on to have an attack with appropriate EEG changes.

Photic stimulation. Exposure to light flickering at 4–30 flashes per second or more normally produces rhythmic EEG activity at the flash rate, termed photic following. Anomalous responses are often observed, for instance following at a harmonic of the flash frequency, or irregular posterior slow activity; some of these are genetically determined but of no clinical significance. Less commonly, generalized epileptiform discharges are elicited by flicker, most readily at about 18 flashes per second. These may be self-sustaining and continue for some hundreds of milliseconds or longer after stimulation has ceased; in susceptible subjects continued photic stimulation will give rise to an overt seizure. Some authors attach the term 'photosensitivity' to all anomalous photic responses, whereas others confine it to the triggering of generalized spike-and-wave activity (the 'photoconvulsive response' of Bickford and co-workers (1952)). However defined, photosensitivity is genetically determined and is considerably more common in children than in adults. Some 20% of children with epilepsy show a self-sustaining photoconvulsive response. The diagnostic specificity of this phenomenon is disputed; various authors have reported photosensitivity in as many as 15% of normal children but have generally failed clearly to distinguish between photoconvulsive and other anomalous responses.

Photosensitivity in a child with epilepsy has practical significance. It tends to support the classification of the epilepsy as idiopathic and may justify the screening of siblings for possible seizure disorders. More importantly, in some 50% of photosensitive children with epilepsy, all attacks are apparently triggered by visual stimuli and no spontaneous seizures occur. In such patients it may be possible to prevent attacks without the use of drugs, simply by avoidance of provocative stimuli. As many as 30% of children with photosensitive epilepsy may use visual stimuli to induce seizures. Some children, often mentally handicapped, induce attacks by waving the outspread fingers of one hand in front of the eyes while gazing at a bright light. A more common and less easily recognized manoeuvre involves a slow eye-closure with lid fluttering, itself easily mistaken for a seizure or tic. EEG and video monitoring in a well-lit environment may help to prove the occurrence of self-induction, and should be considered in any therapy-resistant photosensitive child.

Sleep. Sleep has a marked effect on epilepsy, and some patients have seizures only in sleep or immediately after wakening. In general, epileptiform phenomena, particularly focal discharges, occur most readily in sleep. Recording during sleep, induced by sedative drugs or prolonged wakefulness, therefore plays an important role in the EEG investigation of epilepsy.

THE EEG AND CLASSIFICATION OF THE EPILEPSIES

Various specific epileptic syndromes are recognized within a more general classification of the epilepsies (Commission on Classification and Terminology of the International League Against Epilepsy, 1989). The epilepsies are divided in two dimensions. First, a distinction is made between 'generalized' epilepsies in which seizures apparently arise simultaneously in both hemispheres, and 'partial' (or 'localization-related') epilepsies in which seizure onset is confined to a discrete region of cortex. The second dimension distinguishes symptomatic epilepsies in patients with structural brain disease, cryptogenic epilepsies due to presumed but unproven pathology, and idiopathic epilepsies arising in a structurally normal brain. These features are reflected in the EEG, which therefore serves as a valuable aid to classification.

In *idiopathic generalized epilepsies* both ictal and interictal discharges are conventionally described as generalized. In fact, they usually show a frontal emphasis, as typified by the bilateral spike-and-wave activity in absences, and may exhibit minor asymmetries. Ongoing activity is usually essentially normal.

By contrast, in *symptomatic generalized epilepsies* there is usually a diffuse abnormality of ongoing EEG activity, reflecting the generalized cerebral pathology. Interictal epileptiform discharges are generally of varied topography, both multifocal and generalized. Several different seizure types may occur in any one patient and ictal EEG findings are correspondingly varied.

The *idiopathic partial epilepsies* are virtually confined to the various forms of benign childhood epilepsy, characterized by conspicuous interictal centrotemporal sharp waves in the most common variant (benign childhood epilepsy with Rolandic spikes) and by posterior spike-and-wave discharges in the rarer occipital form.

Symptomatic partial epilepsies are characterized by focal discharges, both at seizure onset and in the interictal state. These are not, however, always visible in the scalp EEG (see section on Long-term EEG monitoring below), although they are readily demonstrable by intracranial recording in those few patients in whom this procedure is carried out before surgical treatment. Partial seizures and ictal or interictal focal discharges may propagate to involve the homologous region of the contralateral hemisphere, or may become generalized. If secondary generalization occurs rapidly, the underlying focal phenomena (both clinical and electrographic) may be difficult to identify, leading to possible misdiagnosis. Localized interictal abnormalities of ongoing activity may be present, reflecting either the causative pathology or a functional disturbance due to the seizures themselves.

These EEG features are found most consistently in epilepsies arising in the temporal lobes. Interictal discharges may be propagated from mesial temporal structures to appear over the anterior temporal region. If the seizures originate in lateral temporal neocortex the discharges are more likely to have a mid-temporal maximum. Background asymmetries, especially in respect of fast activity, are common. In partial epilepsies of extra-temporal origin, focal epileptiform discharges may be less in evidence. Particularly in mesiobasal frontal epilepsies, interictal EEG discharges may be absent or seen only as secondarily generalized spike-and-wave activity.

Surprisingly, perhaps, the ictal EEGs of patients with partial epilepsies do not always show localizing features. Complex partial seizures of temporal lobe origin may be accompanied in the EEG by bilateral rhythmic θ activity, and simple partial seizures, particularly those with psychic or viscerosensory symptoms, may produce no visible EEG change. Seizures arising in the peri-Rolandic region may produce focal spikes over the appropriate area, but here too, if the ictal symptoms are brief and anatomically restricted, ictal EEG changes may be absent. Ictal recording during seizures of mesial or orbital frontal origin presents particular diagnostic difficulties. Rhythmic bilateral or unilateral frontal slow activity may be seen, but is readily mistaken for eye-movement artefact.

SPECIFIC EPILEPSY SYNDROMES OF CHILDHOOD AND ADOLESCENCE

Within the general classification of the epilepsies, various specific epilepsy syndromes are distinguished, all of which are characterized by a particular age of onset within the period from infancy to adolescence. Most present more or less distinctive EEG features.

Neonatal epilepsies

It is generally acknowledged that the present classification of neonatal epilepsies is incomplete, but the following are recognized by the International League Against Epilepsy (ILAE).

Benign idiopathic neonatal convulsions ('fifth-day fits') are partial seizures with clonus and apnoea occurring in otherwise healthy full-term infants. There is a prompt response to medication, and subsequent development is normal. Interictal EEG findings include generalized or multifocal discharges, but typically sharp waves occurring in bursts over the central regions ('théta pointu alternant') in 60% (Dehan et al, 1977). During seizures, rhythmic spikes or slow waves are seen without postictal suppression.

Benign familial neonatal convulsions comprise clonic or apnoeic attacks developing on the second or third day of life. This rare familial condition shows dominant inheritance. No specific EEG pattern is known; the record may be normal or abnormal.

Early myoclonic encephalopathy presents in the neonatal period or early infancy with erratic myoclonias shifting from one part of the body to another (Aicardi and Goutières, 1978). The interictal EEG shows generalized irregular polyspike and wave discharges against a background comprising bursts of slow activity with intervening periods of low-amplitude mixed fast and slow components. The pattern may evolve to atypical hypsarrhythmia (see below).

Other proposed neonatal syndromes not included in the ILAE classification include the following.

Unilateral neonatal status epilepticus develops before the sixth day, with stereotyped partial seizures. The EEG shows localized discharges and interictal background abnormalities. Prognosis is determined by the pathology.

Severe cryptogenic neonatal status epilepticus is seen from first 5 days of life up to 6 weeks. The EEG shows sustained high-voltage activity interrupted by brief periods of partial suppression; bursts of α frequency may occur during or following seizures.

Tonic spasms, with extension of the limbs, have a poor prognosis because they frequently accompany intraventricular haemorrhage. The EEG becomes desynchronized and reduced in amplitude during attacks.

Early infantile encephalopathy (Ohtahara, 1978) presents at a few days of age after a normal delivery, with flexor or extensor spasms, increasing in frequency over days or weeks. The EEG shows a suppression–burst pattern which may be unilateral or bilateral, but asynchronous. The tonic spasms are accompanied by an electrodecremental event in the EEG.

The currently recognized syndromes account for a minority of attacks occurring in the neonatal period, some types of which have not been conclusively shown to be epileptic in nature. Mizrahi (1987) suggests that a major consideration is the presence or absence of ictal EEG changes. Focal clonic and tonic attacks are consistently accompanied by discharges and are clearly epileptic. However, myoclonias occur both with and without EEG discharges and there are probably both epileptic and non-epileptic forms. No EEG change is seen during generalized tonic posturing nor with various stereotyped quasi-voluntary behaviours termed 'subtle' seizures. These can often be elicited by stimulation or postural changes and inhibited by physical restraint. These attacks are probably of non-epileptic origin.

Syndromes after the neonatal period

The recognized epileptic syndromes of later infancy, childhood and adolescence are described below.

West's syndrome (infantile spasms) presents a characteristically disorganized EEG pattern termed 'hypsarrhythmia'. This comprises generalized high-voltage irregular slow activity intermixed with multifocal spikes and sharp waves. The topography of the discharges is inconsistent and the overall picture chaotic. The ictal EEG usually shows an electro-decremental event, often with fast activity and preceded by a high-voltage slow wave with or without a spike. In some patients there is a different ictal pattern with high-amplitude slow waves and spikes. Occassionally, hypsarrhythmia is unilateral. The hypsarrhythmic EEG, although characteristic, is not inseparable from the syndrome. Some patients with infantile spasms fail to show hypsarrhythmia (and generally have a more favourable prognosis); others may show the typical EEG without salaam attacks. A rapid clinical and EEG response to adrenocorticotrophic hormone is a favourable sign, and EEG improvement usually precedes clinical change.

Febrile convulsions fall outside the formal definition of epilepsy as they do not represent a liability to spontaneous recurring seizures. However, as a small minority of patients (particularly those with prolonged or unilateral seizures) do subsequently develop epilepsy the diagnosis may be confidently established only by hindsight. After brief bilateral febrile convulsions the risk of subsequent epilepsy is not more than 5%, and it might be hoped that the EEG would be of prognostic value. Unfortunately this is not the case. Postictal slowing of background activity reflects the length of the seizure, and epileptiform discharges may occur in the first few days after a convulsion. These features are of little value for predicting the subsequent development of epilepsy. The EEG may, however, serve a role in identifying acute cerebral disease such as encephalitis, underlying both the seizure and the pyrexia.

The *Lennox–Gastaut syndrome* is a symptomatic or cryptogenic generalized epilepsy of mid-childhood, characterized by atonic and axial tonic seizures, and less consistently associated with atypical absences, myoclonic jerks and generalized tonic–clonic as well as partial seizures. The EEG is usually grossly abnormal with diffuse background slowing and multifocal and generalized discharges, as might be expected in a severe symptomatic generalized epilepsy. Slow spike-and-wave EEG activity (at less than 2.5 cycles/s) is seen and is one of the diagnostic criteria of the syndrome.

Benign myoclonic epilepsy in infancy presents after 6 months of age with isolated myoclonic seizures. The EEG shows sporadic spike-and-wave discharges in waking which increase during sleep.

Severe myoclonic epilepsy in infancy shows a more florid picture with generalized clonic and myoclonic seizures, partial seizures and atypical absences. Early in the condition the EEG may be normal but later fast generalized spike-and-wave and focal abnormalities appear.

It has been disputed whether *myoclonic astatic epilepsy of early childhood* is distinct from a mild cryptogenic form of the Lennox–Gastaut syndrome. It presents in late infancy or the early preschool period, usually with generalized tonic–clonic seizures. The interictal EEG is normal at first or contains excess θ activity. Later, when myoclonic and astatic seizures appear, there is irregular fast spike-and-wave activity, and often photosensitivity.

Childhood absence epilepsy presents at 6–7 years, with absences but without myoclonus. The EEG contains regular 3 cycles/s spike-and-wave activity against a normal background. Rhythmic posterior δ activity may occur.

Epilepsy with myoclonic absences is similar to the above but the seizures are accompanied by myoclonus and the prognosis is less favourable. The EEG findings are similar to those in childhood absence epilepsy.

Juvenile absence epilepsy appears later, in the early teens. The EEG shows spike-and-wave activity typically slightly faster than 3 cycles/s.

Benign partial epilepsy of childhood with Rolandic spikes is an idiopathic epilepsy characterized by focal seizures with somatosensory symptoms mainly during sleep. The EEG shows numerous large negative centro-temporal spikes or sharp waves, often with a slow wave. Usually the electrical field of the spike is a dipole with a positivity in the mid-frontal region. Some 20% of patients also show generalized spikes and waves or polyspikes and waves which are activated during slow-wave and REM sleep. All these abnormalities increase during sleep and, particularly in the early stages of the disorder, a sleep recording may be required to demonstrate the typical and virtually diagnostic Rolandic spikes. A liability to this EEG abnormality is genetically determined: some children with Rolandic spikes have no overt seizures; others may show them in the presence of some other idiopathic epilepsy syndrome with multifactorial inheritance.

In *benign partial epilepsy of childhood with occipital foci* there are interictal posterior–temporal–occipital spike-and-wave activity or sharp waves. The seizures are characterized by visual symptoms, nausea and vomiting, and occasionally hemiconvulsions.

Electrical status epilepticus during slow sleep (ESES) presents with progressive cognitive deterioration, associated with, usually infrequent, seizures that are often nocturnal. Only sporadic epileptiform discharges may be seen in the waking EEG; spike-and-wave activity is present during 85% or more of slow-wave sleep but not in REM. EEG recording during deep sleep is essential to establish the diagnosis, which is probably often missed through failure to perform adequate EEG examination.

The *Landau–Kleffner syndrome*, or acquired epileptic aphasia, is a similar condition, also leading to cognitive deterioration but particularly characterized by loss of acquired language skills. Seizures are observed in only two thirds of the patients and are usually infrequent. The waking EEG shows epileptiform activity, not necessarily very abundant, which is usually generalized, or multifocal, often with a variable distribution, but in some cases unilateral. During sleep many patients show ESES.

Chronic progressive epilepsia continua of childhood is due either to a discrete cerebral lesion or to more diffuse Rasmussen's encephalitis. If there is a discrete lesion, focal discharges occur against a normal background. In Rasmussen's encephalitis there are marked diffuse background abnormalities and often bilateral discharges. The encephalitis is usually unilateral and the EEG asymmetrical. Extensive damage to one hemisphere may reduce all EEG activity on that side, so that the discharges are paradoxically of greater amplitude over the unaffected hemisphere.

Juvenile myoclonic epilepsy is familial and in most pedigrees studied is due to a genetic defect involving chromosome 6. Typically in the mid-teens, the patient develops irregular bilateral myoclonic jerks occurring mainly within 1 h of wakening. Irregular fast multiple spike-and-wave discharges occur in the interictal EEG and during the myoclonic seizures; many patients are photosensitive.

Epilepsy with generalized tonic–clonic seizures on awakening presents in adolescence but may continue into adult life. The background interictal EEG activity is often abnormal and generalized spike-and-wave discharges occur.

The *progressive myoclonic epilepsies of childhood and adolescence* include various unrelated encephalopathies with the common clinical features of myoclonus, other types of seizure, progressive mental deterioration and variable neurological symptoms. Some of these neurodegenerative conditions have characteristic EEG features. However, in general the EEG shows bursts of spikes, spike-and-wave activity and multiple spikes and slow waves, with slowing of ongoing activity and disruption of sleep patterns.

EEG INVESTIGATION OF CHILDREN WITH EPILEPSY

The EEG is over-used, under-used and mis-used for the assessment of possible seizure disorders. It is over-used as an aid to the essentially clinical diagnosis of epilepsy, which it can in general only support and rarely exclude. It is under-used as a means of answering specific questions, for instance concerning classification of epilepsy or the possible occurrence of brief seizures that are hard to detect by unaided clinical observation. It is mis-used as a method of assessing clinical progress and prognosis. In children the EEG is particularly mis-used as a screening test for epilepsy when there are thought to be 'soft signs' of organic cerebral disease, or episodic behaviours that could possibly be ictal in nature.

The main use of the EEG in paediatric epileptology is for identifying syndromes rather than for establishing, or excluding, epilepsy. Thus, slow spike-and-wave activity is a diagnostic criteria for the Lennox–Gastaut syndrome, and ESES is essentially an EEG diagnosis. Although possibly a reflection on standards of history taking, in practice benign childhood epilepsy is often identified by the finding of Rolandic spikes, and juvenile myoclonic epilepsy by the characteristic multiple spike-and-wave discharges. If, in a particular clinical context, the EEG excludes the only plausible syndrome, another diagnosis should be considered. For instance, if a child reported to be inattentive overbreathes for 3 min hard enough to produce EEG slowing, and does not exhibit spike-and-wave activity, active absence epilepsy can be excluded and some other explanation should be sought.

A more individualized problem-solving approach to the use of the EEG in epilepsy often requires that recording be undertaken during seizures; this, in turn, demands prolonged EEG monitoring, which is considered below.

Long-term EEG monitoring

As the clinical and electrophysiological manifestations of epilepsy are inter-mittent, a routine EEG recording of some 30 min duration will often fail to show epileptiform activity, which may indeed occur only during seizures. Conversely, interictal discharges may be of doubtful clinical significance. As noted above, epileptiform activity occurs in many patients with cerebral disease but without known seizures. Thus frequent spikes in the EEG of a brain-damaged mentally handicapped child with an episodic disturbance of behaviour do not indicate that this is ictal in nature. Finally, even if seizures are documented in the EEG laboratory this offers little evidence of their frequency and significance in daily life.

These and similar problems can be addressed by long-term simultaneous monitoring of EEG and behaviour. In hospital, the EEG can be monitored over some days by *telemetry* and behaviour documented by video recording. Alternatively, *ambulatory monitoring* of the EEG can be carried out in the patient's everyday environment with a portable cassette recorder, but under these conditions behavioural documentation is less reliable and usually depends on reports of carers. These two technologies have different applications.

Telemetry

The restriction of activity required to obtain a routine EEG recording will be tolerated by a lively child for only a limited period. Moreover, whilst a child remains still on a chair or couch it may be impossible to detect subtle ictal phenomena or the effects of behaviour and environment on seizures. Telemetry allows the EEG to be recorded through a long flexible cable or by a radio link. The patient must remain within the restricted environment of a single room or telemetry suite, but can engage in a range of sedentary activities sufficient to prevent boredom and to allow behavioural changes to be observed.

Documentation of behaviour by video recording is essential. Subtle ictal events may be recognized only when the EEG is compared with behaviour. Thus a momentary hesitation in speech or arrest of activity may be identified as ictal because of a consistent relationship to an EEG change. Conversely, EEG discharges which appear to be subclinical may be found to be consistently accompanied by subtle behavioural events, which must be regarded as seizures.

Interpretation of telemetric findings can be difficult or equivocal, particularly when a supposed ictal clinical event occurs without apparent EEG change. By definition, an epileptic seizure is due to abnormal neuronal activity, but this may not be evident in the EEG recorded from the scalp. Abnormal activity in small or deep neuronal populations may not be reflected at all in the EEG, or may produce, not spiky epileptiform activity, but rather minor changes in ongoing rhythms. Various different seizure types are fairly consistent in this respect. Absences, for instance, are consistently accompanied by spike-and-wave discharges; a brief behavioural arrest without such an EEG signature is, unequivocally, not an absence. Some seizures are usually or often associated with non-epileptiform EEG changes. Examples include low-amplitude fast activity during tonic seizures, an electrodecremental event during an infantile spasm or an atonic seizure, and bitemporal θ activity during many complex partial seizures. Simple partial seizures, particularly with psychic or viscerosensory symptoms, are most likely to produce no EEG change. Interpretation of an apparently negative ictal EEG thus depends on the nature of the seizure and correlation in time of the electrical and behavioural recording to detect subtle EEG changes.

Ambulatory monitoring

An ambulatory recorder is light and compact; it can be carried by a child on a shoulder-strap or waistband and used outside the hospital environment. The EEG is registered on a standard audio-cassette which runs continuously at a low tape speed for 24 h. Intervention is required at least once daily to change the tape and batteries and to check the electrodes. Despite continuing technical development, the quality of the recording is limited by the storage capacity of the cassette and is inferior to that of telemetry. This increases the difficulty of identifying subtle changes and of distinguishing EEG activity from the artefacts produced by an actively moving child. Systems exist for synchronous video recording but are little used and tend to defeat the object of allowing unrestricted movement. Behaviour is therefore generally documented by carers and cannot be accurately synchronized with the EEG.

Ambulatory monitoring is not a substitute for telemetry in detecting minor seizures, locating ictal onset or deciding whether subtle events are epileptic. It is, however, the preferred method for investigating a known EEG phenomenon in a particular everyday setting, for instance to determine the frequency of absence seizures in class.

Use of the EEG in diagnosis of childhood epilepsies

Some typical scenarios will be briefly considered.

'Routine' investigation of newly diagnosed epilepsy

The EEG is chiefly of value to identify the syndrome, with implications for management and prognosis. Usually only routine interictal records are obtained at this stage of assessment. The normality or abnormality of ongoing activity, and the presence or absence of localized changes, may provide some guide to the classification of the suspected epilepsy. However, the EEG is likely to be of much greater value for classification and will incidentally provide some confirmation of the diagnosis of epilepsy if epileptiform discharges can be captured. As indicated above, those epileptiform phenomena that are relevant to the diagnosis of epilepsy can be confused with spiky waveforms which occur in normal subjects. This confusion exists not only in routine practice but also in the literature, and it is difficult to find large reliable studies of the prevalence of epileptiform activity, defined according to clear criteria, in populations with and without epilepsy. Some such data exist for adults (for a review see Binnie, 1992) but are less readily available for children.

Repeated EEG investigation of adults with epilepsy suggests that approximately one third consistently exhibit epileptiform activity in the waking interictal EEG, one sixth never do so, and the remaining half show discharges in about one third of routine records and not in the others (Ajmone Marsan and Zivin, 1970). Thus a single waking EEG will demonstrate epileptiform activity in about 50% of adults with epilepsy. Repeated investigation will eventually demonstrate discharges in 85%, that is in all but those patients who never show them in the interictal waking state. However, sleep recording will immediately provide a yield of some 80% and should arguably be performed as part of the initial EEG investigation of all patients with suspected epilepsy. There remain some 8% of adults in whom repeated wake-and-sleep records fail to demonstrate epileptiform activity. If any of these present a clinical problem that requires EEG evidence, long-term monitoring will usually be the next step. The specificity of epileptiform activity to epilepsy is also difficult to establish. Some 3% of patients with non-epileptic organic cerebral or psychiatric disorders exhibit epileptiform EEG activity (Zivin and Marsan, 1968; Bridgers, 1987), but its prevalence is an order of magnitude less in large series of neurologically screened healthy adults such as aircrew (Robin et al, 1978; Gregory et al, 1993). Comparable statistics for children, with adequate neurological assessment and clearly defined criteria of EEG assessment, do not appear to be available. The prevalence of epileptiform activity in children with and without epilepsy is reported, probably correctly, to be greater than in adults.

Although the main role of the EEG is in classification, and to a lesser degree in confirmation, of epilepsy, routine examination often yields other clinically significant, unexpected findings. The discovery of unsuspected photosensitivity or frequent brief unrecognized seizures, for instance, may be of considerable practical importance. The possibility of obtaining crucial clinical information by serendipity may justify 'routine' EEG investigation of newly diagnosed patients, even where the fact and classification of epilepsy are beyond doubt.

Screening of children with an increased risk or doubtful evidence of epilepsy

In the absence of clear clinical evidence of a seizure disorder, unequivocally abnormal EEG findings should be interpreted with caution and minor anomalies with scepticism. Spiky EEG phenomena unrelated to epilepsy (6 and 14 per second positive spikes, for instance) should be ignored. Rolandic spikes, photosensitivity and regular 3 per second generalized spike-and-wave activity may reflect a genetic liability, rather than an active seizure disorder. However, such findings often justify further enquiry, which may, for instance, reveal previously unrecognized seizures, ictal events related to visual stimuli, myoclonus in proximity to a television set, self-inducing behaviour, etc.

During apparently subclinical EEG discharges, unexpected ictal events can often be detected (see Investigation of children with interictal discharges below). The finding of subtle but overt seizures, identified by their relationship to EEG discharges, serves at the least to confirm a diagnosis of epilepsy.

Investigation of episodic abnormal behaviour

The only reliable method of establishing that a particular episodic behaviour is epileptic is by demonstrating ictal EEG changes. This applies equally to children with known epilepsy and to those without. The possibility of misinterpreting an interictal EEG abnormality in this context was noted above, and arises particularly in children with learning or attention disorders due to underlying cerebral pathology.

The practicalities of capturing an ictal EEG depend on the frequency, nature and circumstances of occurrence of the episodes. It must be recognized, however, that even intensive monitoring may not solve the problem. If the episodic abnormal behaviour is infrequent, there may be little chance of observing it during an acceptable period of monitoring. If it occurs only in specific situations, it may not be seen in the environment of the telemetry laboratory, and ambulatory monitoring will be necessary, which in turn reduces the reliability of behavioural documentation. Again, it should be noted that some types of seizure do not produce ictal EEG changes. In practice, EEG investigation of this problem is difficult, often inconclusive, and unrewarding, unless the patients to be investigated are selected carefully.

Investigation of children with interictal discharges

In many children with few seizures, indeed in some children without manifest epilepsy, frequent epileptiform discharges may be seen in the interictal EEG. If the child sits upright with outstretched arms during recording, momentary loss of muscle tone may be shown to accompany the discharges. Such brief episodes of atonia are strictly epileptic seizures; whether they require treatment will depend on various clinical considerations.

Even in the absence of overt motor changes, if the child performs a task requiring some psychological effort during EEG recording it may be possible to detect brief decrements of performance accompanying apparently subclinical discharges. Appropriate formal psychological tests are available for demonstrating such transitory cognitive impairment (TCI) (Binnie et al, 1987), but often simple *ad hoc* methods such as finger counting may suffice, and these can be applied routinely by the technician in any child found to have subclinical discharges in the alert state. Episodes of TCI are technically epileptic seizures, and may have clinical implications, particularly in a child with learning difficulties. Here, the question may arise of possible medication to suppress the discharges. The practice of 'EEG cosmetics' is rightly deplored but, when a child with psychosocial problems exhibits TCI on psychological testing during EEG recording, there may be a case for a trial of treatment. One controlled trial (Marston et al, 1993) suggested that in such children reduction of discharges by antiepileptic drugs may improve psychosocial function. Criteria for treatment are not yet established, and an important consideration is that drugs do not readily suppress discharges and may themselves cause cognitive deficits.

Investigation of possible epilepsy with mental handicap

As noted previously, epileptiform EEG activity is not uncommon in children with cerebral pathology, even in the absence of any seizure disorder. It is therefore especially important that uncorroborated EEG findings should not be taken as evidence of epilepsy in children with mental handicap. In addition to a generally increased prevalence of epileptiform activity and epilepsy in children with brain damage, cerebral palsy for instance, epilepsy occurs specifically as a feature of some forms of mental handicap and neurodegenerative disorders.

In Down's syndrome, infantile spasms may occur, together with a typical hypsarrhythmic EEG. Other types of epilepsy are not as uncommon in Down's syndrome as was once supposed, and in particular reflex seizures may occur (Guerrini et al, 1990).

The EEG in Angelman's syndrome may contain epileptiform activity which increases to become almost continuous during periods when the child is withdrawn, suggesting that this state represents a non-convulsive status epilepticus.

Epileptiform activity is also found over the centrotemporal regions in Rett's syndrome, particularly during sleep. It occurs both in girls with seizures and in those without. The discharges may be related to the continuous hand movements, and in some children they can be elicited by tapping on the patient's fingers (Robb et al, 1989).

CONCLUSION

Most diagnostic investigations are open to abuse, but none more so than the EEG. One must deplore equally its use as a routine screen to 'exclude epilepsy' or conversely as a last resort to establish epilepsy as the cause of unexplained symptoms in the absence of any other evidence of a seizure disorder. However, as a means of addressing specific issues such as classification, or solving complex problems such as a possible relationship between cognitive difficulties and subclinical discharges, the EEG is an essential aid to the care of children with epilepsy.

REFERENCES

Aicardi J & Goutières F (1978) Encéphalopathie myoclonique néonatale. *Revue d'EEG et de Neurophysiologie* **8:** 99–101.

Ajmone Marsan C & Zivin LS (1970) Factors related to the occurrence of typical paroxysmal abnormalities in the EEG records of epileptic patients. *Epilepsia* **11:** 361–381.

Bickford RG, Sem-Jacobsen CW, White PT & Daly D (1952) Some observations on the mechanism of photic and photo-metrazol activation. *Electroencephalography and Clinical Neurophysiology* **4:** 275–282.

Binnie CD (1992) Electroencephalography. In Laidlaw J, Richens A & Chadwick D (eds) *A Textbook of Epilepsy*, 4th edn, pp 277–278. Edinburgh: Churchill Livingstone.

Binnie CD, Kasteleijn-Nolst Trenité DGA, Smit AM & Wilkins AJ (1987) Interactions of epileptiform EEG discharges and cognition. *Epilepsy Research* **1:** 239–245.

Bridgers SL (1987) Epileptiform abnormalities discovered on electroencephalographic screening of psychiatric inpatients. *Archives of Neurology* **44:** 312–316.

Commission on Classification and Terminology of the International League Against Epilepsy (1989) Proposal for revised classification of epilepsies and epileptic syndromes. *Epilepsia* **30:** 389–399.

Dehan M, Quillerou D, Navelet V et al (1977) Les convulsions du cinquième jour de vie: un nouveau syndrome? *Archives Françaises de Pédiatrie* **34:** 730–742.

Dement W & Kleitman N (1957) Cyclic variations in EEG during sleep and their relation to eye movements, body motility, and dreaming. *Electroencephalography and Clinical Neurophysiology* **9:** 673–690.

Doose H & Gerken H (1973) On the genetics of EEG-anomalies in childhood: IV. Photoconvulsive reaction. *Neuropaediatrie* **4:** 162–171.

Dümermuth G (1968) Variance spectra of electroencephalograms in twins—a contribution to the problem of quantification of EEG background activity in childhood. In Kellaway P & Petersén I (eds) *Clinical Electroencephalography of Children*, pp 119–154. Stockholm: Almquist and Wiksell.

Gloor P, Kalabay O & Giard N (1968) The electroencephalogram in diffuse encephalopathies: electroencephalographic correlates of grey and white matter lesions. *Brain* **91:** 779–802.

Gregory RP, Oates T & Merry RTG (1993) Electroencephalogram epileptiform abnormalities in candidates for aircrew training. *Electroencephalography and Clinical Neurophysiology* **86:** 75–77.

Guerrini R, Genton P, Bureau M et al (1990) Reflex seizures are frequent in patients with Down's syndrome and epilepsy. *Epilepsia* **31:** 406–417.

Lennox WG, Gibbs EL & Gibbs FA (1945) The brain wave pattern, an hereditary trait. Evidence from 74 'normal' pairs of twins. *Journal of Heredity* **36:** 233–243.

Marston D, Besag F, Binnie CD & Fowler M (1993) Effects of transitory cognitive impairment on psychosocial functioning in children with epilepsy: a therapeutic trial. *Developmental Medicine and Child Neurology* **35:** 574–581.

Mizrahi EM (1987) Neonatal seizures: problems in diagnosis and classification. *Epilepsia* **28 (supplement 1):** 546–555.

Ohtahara S (1978) Clinico-electrical delineation of epileptic encephalopathies in childhood. *Asian Medicine* **21:** 7–17.

Robb SA, Harden A & Boyd SG (1989) Rett syndrome: an EEG study in 52 girls. *Neuropediatrics* **20:** 192–195.

Robin JJ, Tolan GD & Arnold JW (1978) Ten-year experience with abnormal EEGs in asymptomatic adult males. *Aviation Space and Environmental Medicine* **49:** 732–736.

Stassen HH, Lykken DT, Propping P & Bomben G (1988) Genetic determination of the human EEG. *Human Genetics* **80:** 165–176.

Steriade M, Gloor P, Llinas RR et al (1990) Basic mechanisms of cerebral rhythmic activities. *Electroencephalography and Clinical Neurophysiology* **76:** 481–508.

Vogel F (1958) *Über die Erblichkeit des normalen EEG. Zwillingsuntersuchungen*. Stuttgart: Thieme.

Zivin L & Ajmone Marsan C (1968) Incidence and prognostic significance of 'epileptiform' activity in the EEG of non-epileptic subjects. *Brain* **91:** 751–778.

Index

Note: Page numbers of article titles are in **bold** type.

Abnormal behaviour, episodic, 602
Absence epilepsy, 461, 478
  EEG, 596–597
Absence seizures, 569
Acquired aphasia, 478
ACTH, 478
Adrenoleukodystrophy, 492
Aicardi syndrome, 492, 541
Ambulatory EEG monitoring, 600
Angelman syndrome, 494, 603
Animal studies, 489–490
Antiepileptic drugs, 464–466, 499, 516–519,
    570–571
  availability of, 465–466
  duration of, 465
  failure of, 519
Antipyretic therapy, 553
Aphasia, acquired, 478
Aspartame, 531
Aura, 567
Automatism, 472, 567
Autosomal single-gene defects—
  dominant, 490–491
  recessive, 491

Behavioural therapy, 538–539
Benign familial neonatal convulsions, 476,
    495
  EEG in, 595
Benign idiopathic neonatal convulsions, 476
  EEG of, 594
Benign myoclonic epilepsy, 477
Benign partial epilepsy, 463
  adolescent, 480
  with occipital paroxysms, 479
  Rolandic, *see under* Rolandic epilepsy
Bett's technique, 539–540
Biofeedback, 538
Blood tests, 548
Brain damage, 549–550, 572
Brain scans, 464, 515, 548–549
  computed tomography, 464, 515, 549–
    550
  MRI, 464, 515, 549–550

Calcium ATPase, 490
Carbamazepine, 405, 517, 570, 571
Care provision, 467
Cerebral tumours, 480
Chinese medicine, 539
Chromosomal disorders, 492
Classification, of epilepsy, 463–464, **471–484**
  by (clinical) history, 463–464
  by computed tomography, 464
  in developing countries, 513
  by EEG, 464, 493–494
  epileptic syndromes (*in chronological order*),
    474–481
    neonatal to 3 months, 475–476
    3 months to 4 years, 476–477
    4 years to 10 years, 478–480
    over 10 years, 480–481
  by MRI, 464
Classification, of seizures, 472–473
Clonazepam, 465, 517
CNS infections, 510–511
CNS tubecular granulomata, 510–511
Cognitive impairment, *see* Mental handicap
Complementary medicine, 539–540
Complex partial epilepsies, 461–462
Complex partial seizures, 473
Computed tomography, 464, 511, 515, 549–
    550
Consanguinity, 512
Convulsions, *see under* Febrile convulsions
    and also Seizures
Costs, in developing countries, 517–518
Counselling, **485–505**
Cross-sectional epidemiological studies, 459
Cryptogenic myoclonic epilepsy, 477
Cryptogenic neonatal status epilepticus, 595

Dahl technique, 539
Developing countries, epilepsy in, **507–527**
  causes of, 510–512
  vs. developed, 508
  diagnosis in, 513–514
    neuro-, 514–515
  epidemiology, 509–510

Developing countries, epilepsy in—(*cont.*)
  prevention of, 522–523
  prognosis, 520–522
  special centres in, 519
  treatment in, 515–519
    counselling, 519–520
  WHO Essential Drug List, 523
Diagnostics, 454–455
  EEG, *see under* EEG
  incorrect, 461–463
  and Munchausen syndrome by proxy, 455
  see also Differential diagnosis, of epilepsy
Diazepam, 465, 517, 552–554
  oral, 554–555
  rectal, 554
    home administration, 554
Diet, 530–531
  ketogenic, 532–536
  oligoantigenic, 536–537
Differential diagnosis, of epilepsy, 461–463
  absence attacks, 461
    in childhood, 461
    myoclonic, 461
  benign partial, 463
  classification of, 463
  complex partial, 461–462
  juvenile myoclonic, 462
  photosensitive, 462
  progressive myoclonic, 462
Dilantin, 461
DNA analysis, 495
Down's syndrome, 492, 603
Drug therapy, 464–466, 516–519, 522–554,
    570–571
  failure, 518–519
  in the fetus, 499

E1 epilepsy mouse, 489–490
Education, 561–566
  failure, 566–572
  of parents, 555–557
EEG, 464, 487–489, 498, 500, 515, 599–600
  age and, 587–588
  epileptiform activity and, 589–591
  febrile seizures, 549
  origin of, 585–586
  pathology and, 588–591
  recording, 586
  telemetry, 599–600
Electrical status epilepticus, during slow sleep
    (ESES syndrome), 479, 597
Epidemiology, of epilepsy, 457–460
  cross-sectional studies, 459
  data for, 458
  developing countries, 509–513
  incidence of, 458
  longitudinal studies, 459–460
  prevalence, 458–459
Epilepsia partialis continua, 480

Epilepsy, in children—
  care and, 467
  classification of, **471–484**, 486, 513, 593–
    594
  complementary medicine and, 539–540
  counselling in, **485–505**, 519–520
    risk assessment, 497–499
  developing countries, centres for, 519–520
  developing countries, epidemiology, **507–
    527**
  diagnosis, 461–463
    in developing countries, 513–514
  drugs for, 464–466
  education and, **561–583**
  epidemiology, 457–460, **507–527**
  febrile convulsions, 457
  febrile seizures, 550–551; *see also under*
    Febrile seizures
  genetic counselling, **485–505**
  history (non-clinical), 452–453
  informing the child, 466
  inheritance of, 486–490
  international classifications, 453–455 463–
    464
  literature on, 468
  misdiagnosis, 454–455; *see also under*
    Differential diagnosis, of epilepsy
  needs and, 452
  neurophysiological investigations, **585–604**
  non-drug approaches, **529–546**
  non-febrile, 457–460
  patterns of, 455–457
  perceptions of, in developing countries,
    512–513
  prevention of, 460, 522–523
  professions and, 466–467
  prognosis, 466, 520–521
  risk, 497–499
  surgery in, 541–544
  treatment, 515–516; *see also* Drug therapy
Epileptiform EEG activity, 589–591
  FIRDA (delta activity), 590
  periodicity, 591
  PLEDs, 591
  slow waves, 591
  theta activity, 590
  triphasic complexes, 591
ESES syndrome, 497, 597
Essential Drug List (WHO), 523
Ethosuximide, 465, 517

Familial neonatal convulsions, benign, 495
Families, 487–489
Fatigue, 568
Febrile convulsions, 457, 596
  inheritance of, 489
Febrile seizures—
  blood tests, 548
  brain damage, 549

brain imaging, 548–549
death from, 549
diagnosis and, 548
epilepsy and, 550–551
identification of, 547–548
lumbar puncture and, 548
management of, 552–555
parents and, 555–557
prevention of, 553–555
    daily basis, 553–554
    pyresis and, 553
treatment with diazepam, 552–555
    oral, 554–555
    rectal, 554
Feldamate, 465
Fetal hydantoin syndrome, 499
Fetal trimethadione syndrome, 499
Fetus, drugs and, 499
Fibre, dietary, 530–531
Flicker-induced epilepsy, 531–532
    see also Photosensitive epilepsy
Focal discharges, 568–569
Fragile X syndrome, 492

Gabapentin, 465
GABA receptors, 496–497
Gaucher's disease, 491
Gender, and mitochondrial inheritance, 493
Generalized epilepsy, and EEG and, 593–594
Generalized-onset epilepsy, 487–488
Genetics, molecular analysis, 495–497
    see also Families and also Inheritance, of
    epilepsies
Generalized seizures, 472
    secondary, 473
Genetic defects, 490–494
    chromosomal, 492
    genomic imprinting, 494
    mitochondrial inheritance, 493
    multifactorial inheritance, 492–493
    single gene, 490–492
        autosomal dominant, 490–491
        autosomal recessive, 491
        X-linked dominant, 492
        X-linked recessive, 492
Genomic imprinting, 494
Grand mal, 478
    on awakening, 481

Haemophilus influenzae, 522
Head traumas, 512
Herbal medicines, 539–540
History (non-clinical), of epilepsy, 452–453
HIV infection, 511
Holism, 538–539
Homoeopathy, 539–540
'Hot-water epilepsy', 512
Huntington's disease, 491, 492, 494
Hydantoin, see Phenytoin

Hyperventilation, 592
Hyssop, 539

Ias gene, 490
Immunization, 522
Impulsive petit mal, 488
Infantile encephalitis, 595
Infantile epileptic encephalopathy, 476
Infantile spasms, see West's syndrome
Infections, 522–523
    see also specific forms of
Inheritance, of epilepsies, 486–490
    animal studies, 489–490
    classification studies, 486
    epidemiological studies, 486–487
    family studies, 487–489
        generalized onset, 487–488
        partial epilepsy, 488–489
    febrile convulsions, 489
    multifactorial, 492–493
Intellectual impairment, see Mental handicap
    and also Brain damage
Interictal discharges, EEG, 602–603
Interictal psychoses, 568
International Classification of Epilepsy and
    Epileptic Syndromes, 473–474

Juvenile myoclonic epilepsy (Janz syndrome),
    462, 480, 488, 496, 597–598

Kearns–Sayre syndrome, 493
Ketogenic diets, 532–536
Kuf's disease, 491

Lafora disease, 491
Lamotrigine, 465, 570
Landau-Kleffner syndrome, 478, 541, 597
Lennox–Gastaut syndrome, 474, 477, 542,
    571, 596
Leach–Nyhan disease, 492
Light flickering, 462, 478, 532, 592–593
Linkage analysis, 495–497
Literature, on epilepsy, 468
Longitudinal epidemiological studies, 459–
    460
Lowe's oculocerebrorenal syndrome, 492
Lumbar puncture, 548

MCT diets, see Triglycerides, dietary
MELAS syndrome, 493
Menke's syndrome, 492
Mental handicap, 572–576, 603
Mitochondrial inheritance, 493
Molecular genetics analysis, 495–497
    linkage analysis (random markers), 495–497
        benign familial neonatal convulsions, 495
    genes involved, 496–497
    juvenile myoclonic epilepsy, 496
    Unverricht–Lundborg, 496

MRI, 464, 515, 549–550
Munchausen syndrome by proxy, 455
Myoclonic absence attacks, 461
Myoclonic absences, epilepsy with, 478
Myoclonic-astatic EEG, 596
Myoclonic encephalopathy, EEG, 595–597
Myoclonic epilepsy, 462, 496, 551, 595–598
    benign, 477
    juvenile, *see* Juvenile myoclonic epilepsy
        (Janz syndrome)
    myoclonic absences, 461
    progressive (Unverricht–Lundborg), 462,
        496
    severe, 477
        astatic, 477
        cryptogenic, 477

Neonatal convulsions, 495
Neonatal epilepsy, 594–595
Neonatal seizures, 455–456
    causes, 456
    congenital, 456
    drug-induced, 456
    infections and, 456
    post-natal, 456–457
Neuronal ceroid lipofuscinosis, 491
Nitrazepam, 465, 517
Nocturnal focal Rolandic epilepsy, 463
    see also Rolandic epilepsy
Non-convulsive status epilepticus, 569–570
Non-febrile epilepsy, 457–460
    cross-sectional studies of, 459
    incidence of, 458
    information needs and, 458
    longitudinal studies and, 459–460
    prevalence of, 458–459

Oligoantigenic diets, 536–537
Oxycarbamazepine, 465

Parasitic infections, 511
Parents, and febrile seizures, 555–557
Partial epilepsies, 461–463
    adolescent, 480
    benign, 463
        with centrotemporal spikes, *see* Rolandic
        epilepsy
    complex, 461–462
    EEG of, 593–594
    inheritance of, 488–489
    secondary (symptomatic), 479–480
Partial seizures, 472–473
    automatisms, 472
    complex, 473
    simple, 473
Petit mal, 488
Phenobarbitone, 465–466, 553
Phenylketonuria, 491
Phenytoin, 465, 495, 517, 553–554, 570

Photic stimulation, 462, 532, 592–593
Photosensitive epilepsy, 462, 488, 532, 592–593
Postictal changes, 567–568
Postnatal seizures, 456–457
    and neonatal, 455–456
Post-neonatal seizures, 456–457
Prader–Willi syndrome, 494
Pregnancy, 499
Primary epileptic syndromes, 474
Primidone, 465
Prodrome, 567
Professional advice, 466–467
Progressive myoclonic epilepsy, 462
Pyridoxine deficiency, *see* Vitamin B$_6$
    deficiency

Ramsay Hunt syndrome, 491
Rasmussen's syndrome, 480, 541, 571, 597
Recurrent febrile seizures, 550–551
Restriction fragment length polymorphisms,
    495
Rett's syndrome, 603
Risks, in epilepsy, 497–499
    assessment of, 497–499
    empiric, 498–499
        offspring, 498–499
        sibling, 498
    fetal, drugs and, 499
Rolandic discharges, 488
Rolandic epilepsy, 463, 479, 597

Schooling, 571
    special, 579–580
    teasing and, 571
Secondary epileptic syndromes, 474
Seizures—
    generalized, 472
    genuine, non-epileptic, 455
    neonatal, 455–456
    partial, 472–473
    postnatal, 456–457
    see also specific forms of and also Febrile
        convulsions
Sibling risk, 498
Simple partial seizures, 473
Skull cap (*Scutellaria*), 539
Sleep, 463, 479, 567–568, 570, 593
Sodium valproate, 465, 499, 517, 553–554,
    570–571
Special schools, 579–580
Spielmeyer–Vogt disease, 491
Status epilepticus, 595
Stress, 538–539
Subacute sclerosing panencephalitis, 511
Surgery, 541–544, 571

Tay–Sachs disease, 491
Telemetry, 599–600
Television-induced epilepsy, 531–532

see also Photosensitive epilepsy
Time, and epilepsy onset, 475
Trisomy, 492
Tonic–clonic seizures, EEG of, 598
Transitory cognitive impairment, 602–603
Triglycerides, dietary, 534, 536
Trimethadione, 499

Unclassifiable epilepsy, 463
Unverricht–Lundborg epilepsy, 491, 496, 500

Valproate, *see* Sodium valproate
VDUs, 532
    see also Photosensitive epilepsy

Video-telemetry, 538
Vigabatrin, 465, 570
Viral disease, 511
Vitamin B$_6$ deficiency, 476, 491
Vitamins, 530
Voluntary societies, 466

West's syndrome, 474, 476, 595–596
WHO Essential Drug List, 523
Wolf's syndrome, 492

X-linked gene defects, 492
    dominant, 492
    recessive, 492